HOW TO READ PEDIATRIC ECGS

THIRD EDITION

HOW TO READ PEDIATRIC ECGS
THIRD EDITION

MYUNG K. PARK. M.D.
Professor of Pediatrics
Head, Division of Pediatric Cardiology
University of Texas Health Science Center
San Antonio, Texas

WARREN G. GUNTHEROTH, M.D.
Professor of Pediatrics
Head, Division of Pediatric Cardiology
University of Washington School of Medicine
Seattle, Washington

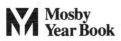
Mosby
Year Book

St. Louis   Baltimore   Boston   Chicago   London   Philadelphia   Sydney   Toronto

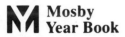

Mosby
Year Book

Dedicated to Publishing Excellence

Sponsoring Editor: Stephanie Manning
Assistant Editor: Jane Petrash
Associate Managing Editor, Manuscript Services: Deborah Thorp
Senior Production Assistant: Maria Nevinger
Proofroom Manager: Barbara Kelly

5 6 7 8 9 0 CL MA 00 99 98 97

Library of Congress Cataloging-in-Publication Data

Park, Myung K. (Myung Kun), 1934-
    How to read pediatric ECGs / Myung K. Park, Warren G. Guntheroth.
    —3rd ed.
        p.   cm.
    Includes bibliographical references and index.
    ISBN 0-8016-6834-4
    1. Electrocardiography—Interpretation.   2. Pediatric cardiology—
Diagnosis.   I. Guntheroth, Warren G.   II. Title.
    [DNLM: 1. Electrocardiography—in infancy & childhood.
2. Vectorcardiography—in infancy & childhood.   WS 290 P235h]
RJ423.5.E43P37 1992
618.92′1207547—dc20   92-6218
DNLM/DLC   CIP
for Library of Congress

Dedication

Dedicated to our wives, Issun and Ellie, and our boys, Douglas, Christopher, and Warren Park, and Kurt, Karl, and Sten Guntheroth

Preface to Third Edition

In the third edition of *How to Read Pediatric ECGs;* important changes have been made throughout the book. Major changes can be found in the chapters on basic measurements, hypertrophy, ventricular conduction disturbances, and arrhythmias, which update and improve the text. Continuing feedback and questions from our students and house staff have helped to determine the extent of this revision. We made a substantial expansion in the correlation of scalar ECGs and vectorcardiography. This correlation has improved the understanding of age-related changes in ECGs from the vectorial point of view. We have rewritten a large portion of the section on supraventricular tachycardia with inclusion of current understanding of reciprocating AV tachycardia and its management. The chapter on systematic approaches has been expanded to include more cases, for a total of 20. The chapter on analysis of arrhythmias and AV conduction disturbances has been rearranged, and some rhythm strips have been replaced with better examples. We believe we have made a major improvement in this edition.

We thank those readers who provided the constructive criticism that led to this new edition. We gratefully acknowledge the staff of the Department of Educational Resources at the University of Texas Health Science Center at San Antonio for their superb art and photographic services. The able secretarial assistance of Mrs. Diane Halim, which made our job easier, is also acknowledged.

Myung K. Park, M.D.
Warren G. Guntheroth, M.D.

Preface to Second Edition

This new edition has major changes in two areas. The first change is the replacement of almost all electrocardiographic (ECG) tracings with records of actual size. In the first edition, the ECG tracings were slightly reduced, making it somewhat difficult to measure intervals and durations accurately. Second we have added a new chapter, "Analysis of Arrhythmias and Atrioventricular Conduction Disturbances." Since monitoring for cardiac arrhythmias has become so widely practiced, the ability to recognize and manage rhythm disturbances is increasingly important to most physicians. We present 50 rhythm tracings for the readers to interpret on their own. In addition to these major changes, we have expanded the chapter on cardiac arrhythmia in order to provide a more advanced level of discussion.

The authors thank those readers who gave constructive suggestions that prompted the new edition. We gratefully acknowledge the Department of Educational Resources, University of Texas Health Science Center at San Antonio, for their superb art and photographic work. We are especially indebted to Mr. Dieter Karkut for his excellent photographic skills and willing cooperation, which have made the new edition a significant improvement over the first edition.

Myung K. Park, M.D.
Warren G. Guntheroth, M.D.

Preface to First Edition

This book was written for those pediatricians, family practitioners, residents, interns, and medical students who want to learn how to read pediatric ECGs but have not found a text that is simple and practical. It provides average values by age, with statistically defined ranges.

A vectorial approach, rather than the conventional "pattern" reading, has been used whenever possible, for a more general understanding of the material. We deliberately avoided basic electrophysiology, since our readers will probably have encountered that in earlier courses and texts. However, when the reader has finished this book, he will know most of the useful aspects of electrophysiology. Similarly, we have chosen clarity and simplicity over lengthy presentations of all sides of any controversies that may exist.

This material has been used by medical students and house staff as a syllabus, and the present book is the result of numerous modifications based on the comments of these individuals. We gratefully acknowledge their contributions.

Myung K. Park, M.D.
Warren G. Guntheroth, M.D.

Contents

List of Frequently Used Abbreviations

ASD	Atrial septal defect
AV	Atrioventricular
BBB	Bundle branch block
CAH	Combined atrial hypertrophy
CVH	Combined ventricular hypertrophy
ECD	Endocardial cushion defect
ECG	Electrocardiogram
LA	Left atrium
LAD	Left axis deviation
LAH	Left atrial hypertrophy
LBBB	Left bundle branch block
LLN	Lower limit of normal
LPL	Left precordial lead
LV	Left ventricular or left ventricle
LVH	Left ventricular hypertrophy
PAC	Premature atrial contraction
PAT	Paroxysmal atrial tachycardia
PDA	Patent ductus arteriosus
PVC	Premature ventricular contraction
QRSi	Initial QRS axis
QRSt	Terminal QRS axis
QTc	Corrected QT interval
RA	Right atrium
RAD	Right axis deviation
RAH	Right atrial hypertrophy
RAVT	Reciprocating AV tachycardia
RBBB	Right bundle branch block
RPL	Right precordial lead
RV	Right ventricular or right ventricle
RVH	Right ventricular hypertrophy
SA	Sinoatrial
SSS	Sick sinus syndrome
SVT	Supraventricular tachycardia
TGA	Transposition of the great arteries
ULN	Upper limit of normal
VCG	Vectorcardiogram
VF	Ventricular fibrillation
VSD	Ventricular septal defect
VT	Ventricular tachycardia
WNL	Within normal limits
WPW	Wolff-Parkinson-White

CHAPTER 1

Basic Measurements

In this chapter we will discuss the calculations and measurements that are necessary for interpreting an electrocardiogram (ECG). Examples are given in each section for in-depth understanding. A vectorial approach has been employed throughout the book.

We will begin with a brief review of a normal cycle of cardiac electrical events. One cardiac cycle is represented by successive wave forms on an electrocardiographic tracing: the P wave, QRS complex, and the T wave (Fig 1–1,A). These waves produce two important intervals (PR and QT) and two segments (PQ and ST).

In normal sinus rhythm the sinoatrial (SA) node is the pacemaker for the entire heart; the SA node impulse depolarizes the right and left atria by contiguous spread, producing the P wave (see Figs 1–1,A, B). When the atrial impulse arrives at the atrioventricular (AV) node, it passes through the node at a much slower velocity (see Table 7–1) than any other part of the heart, producing the PQ interval. Once the electrical impulse reaches the bundle of His,

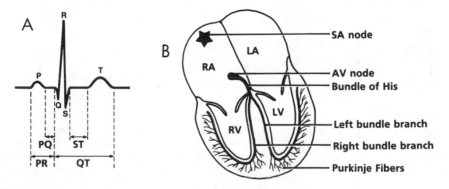

FIG 1–1.
Definition of electrocardiographic configuration **(A),** and diagrammatic representation of conduction system of the heart **(B).**

the conduction velocity becomes very fast and spreads simultaneously down the left and right bundle branches to the ventricular muscle, through the Purkinje fibers, producing the QRS complex. The repolarization of the ventricle produces the T wave, but the repolarization of the atria is not usually visible on the ECG tracing.

HEART RATE

In routine electrocardiographic practice, the recording speed of the paper is 25 mm per second. Therefore,

     1 mm = 0.04 second
     5 mm = 0.20 second (1 large division between the heavy lines)
    25 mm = 1.0 second (5 large divisions)
    30 mm = 1.2 seconds (6 large divisions), and
  300 large divisions = 1 minute

In the top margin of the unmounted ECG paper, every 7.5 cm is marked by a heavy line (Fig 1–2).

           7.5 cm = 3.0 seconds (15 large divisions)

These features are used to determine the heart rate in the following ways:

1. When the heart rate is *fast,* count the RR cycles in 6 large divisions (1.2 seconds) and multiply them by 50. (One can count the RR cycles in 5 large divisions, 1.0 second, and multiply them by 60, but multiplying by 50 is easier than by 60) (Fig 1–3).

2. When the heart rate is *slow,* count the number of large divisions between two R waves and divide into 300 (300 divisions = 1 minute) (Fig 1–4).

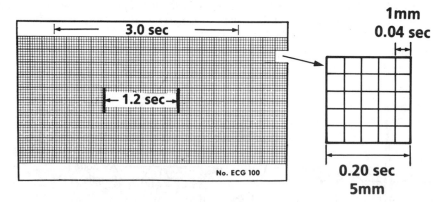

FIG 1–2.
ECG paper. Time is measured on the horizontal axis. Each 1 millimeter equals 0.04 second, and each 5 mm (a large division) equals 0.20 second. Thirty millimeters (or 6 large divisions) equals 1.2 seconds or 1/50 minute. Every 7.5 cm marked on the top margin of the paper equals 3.0 seconds or 1/20 minute.

3. When the tracing is unmounted, count the RR cycles between two markers (3 seconds) on the upper edge of the ECG paper and multiply them by 20 (Fig 1–5).

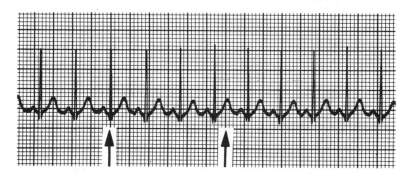

FIG 1–3.
Heart rate of 165 beats per minute. There are about 3.3 cardiac cycles (RR intervals) in 6 large divisions. Therefore, the heart rate is 3.3 × 50 = 165.

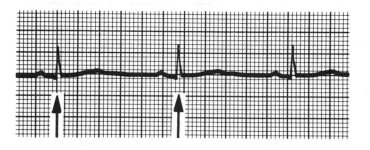

FIG 1–4.
Heart rate of 52 beats per minute. There are 5.8 large divisions between the two arrows. Therefore, the heart rate is 300 ÷ 5.8 = 52.

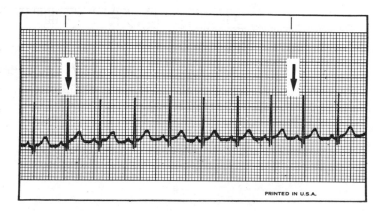

FIG 1–5.
Heart rate of 134 beats per minute. There are about 6.7 cardiac cycles between the two markers (3.0 seconds) in the top margin of the ECG paper. Therefore, the heart rate is 6.7 × 20 = 134.

4. Measure the RR interval directly (seconds), and either
    a. use a table such as Table 3–6 or
    b. divide 60 by the RR interval with a calculator.

In Fig 1–5, the RR interval is 0.44 second ($11 \times 0.04 = 0.44$). Using method 4a, we find from Table 3–6 that when the cycle length (RR interval) is 0.44, the heart rate is approximately 135. Using method 4b the heart rate is 136 ($60 \div 0.44 = 136$).

5. Use a convenient ECG ruler (Fig 1–6). There are many types available.

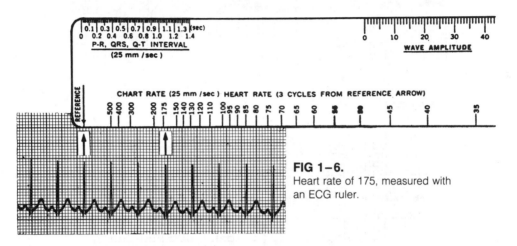

FIG 1–6.
Heart rate of 175, measured with an ECG ruler.

6. Approximation of heart rate can be achieved by memorizing heart rates for selected RR intervals (Fig 1–7). When RR intervals are 5, 10, 15, 20, and 25 mm, the heart rates are 300, 150, 100, 75, and 60 beats per minute, respectively.

FIG 1–7.
Quick method for estimating heart rate.

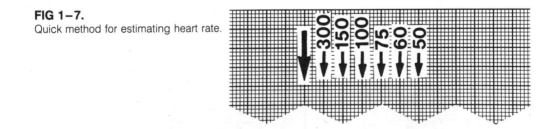

DETERMINATION OF INTERVALS AND DURATIONS

Two intervals (PR and QT) and two durations (P and QRS) are routinely measured (see Fig 1–1,A). The significance of these intervals and durations will be discussed in Chapter 3.

P duration is measured from the onset to the end of the P wave.

PR interval is measured from the onset of the P wave to the beginning of the QRS complex and therefore is sometimes called *PQ interval*. The PR interval is ordinarily measured in lead II or other leads with visible Q waves. In certain leads that are perpendicular to the direction of septal depolarization (which produces a Q wave) the Q wave may be isoelectric or absent. This will result in a longer PR interval (and for the same reason, a shorter QRS duration) than actually exists.

QRS duration is measured from the onset of the Q wave (or R wave if no Q wave is visible) to the termination of the S wave. It is preferable to measure the QRS duration in lead II or in leads with clearly visible Q waves. The QRS duration can be measured in the precordial leads as long as their QRS deflections are small. However, the amplitude of the QRS complex in the precordial leads, such as V2 through V4, is frequently large and the QRS duration will be factitiously prolonged because of the limited frequency response of many direct-writing ECG machines.

QT interval is measured from the onset of the Q wave to the end of the T wave. The same precautions applicable to measuring the PR interval and the QRS duration should be taken in measuring the QT interval; i.e., measure it in leads with visible Q waves.

Measurement of the intervals and durations is expressed in seconds. One should measure either from the left to the left margins (A–B) or from the right to the right margins (A′–B′), because if one measures from the left margin to the right margin (A–B′) or from the right margin to the left margin (A′–B), particularly in the case of the QRS duration, one may obtain artificially prolonged or shortened intervals, depending on the thickness of the line (Fig 1–8). This effect has become less important with newer direct-writing machines which produce thin lines of ECG deflections, but the thickness of such ECG tracings can still affect the measurements of pediatric ECG durations.

FIG 1–8.
Measurements of QRS duration.

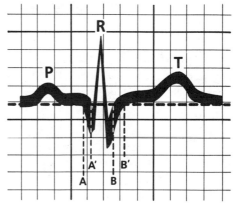

DETERMINATION OF AMPLITUDE

The amplitude of the P wave, QRS complex, and T wave is inspected routinely. The significance of increased or decreased amplitude of each wave form will be discussed in Chapter 3.

The amplitude of any positive deflections, such as P, R, and T waves, is measured from the upper margin of the baseline to the very top of the positive deflection. The amplitude of any negative deflections (Q and S waves) is measured from the lower margin of the baseline to the lowest point of the wave. If a positive deflection is measured from the lower margin of the baseline to the top of the positive deflection (Fig 1–9), a factitiously large amplitude can result, since the baseline itself has a certain thickness. Correct measurement is particularly important in the case of the P amplitude, for which 2.5 mm is considered normal but 3.0 mm is abnormally tall.

Calibration Factor.—"Normal" sensitivity of the ECG is adjusted so that a millivolt signal introduced into the circuit will cause a deflection of 10 mm on the record. The amplitude of ECG deflections is read in millimeters rather than in millivolts. One must check the calibration marker before determining the amplitude of ECG deflections. When the deflections are too big to be recorded, the sensitivity may be reduced to one-half or one-fourth. In case of one-half standardization, the measured height in millimeters should be multiplied by 2 to obtain the correct amplitude of a deflection. With one-fourth standardization, the measured deflection in millimeters should be multiplied by 4 (Fig 1–10).

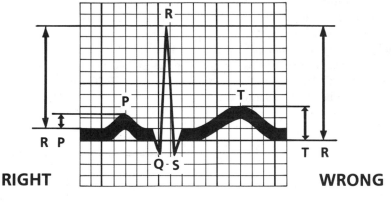

FIG 1–9.
Measurement of amplitude.

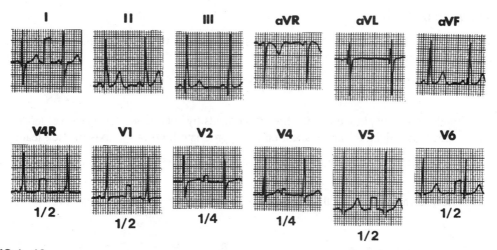

FIG 1–10.
Calibration factors: All the limb leads are recorded on "normal" standardization. The calibration marker shown in lead I indicates that 10 mm deflection is equal to 1 millivolt. The R wave in lead I is 14 mm. The calibration markers for leads V4R, V1, V5, and V6 are in one-half standardization; 5 mm deflection = 1 millivolt. Therefore, the measured amplitude must be multiplied by 2. The R wave in V4R is 32 mm. V2 and V4 are recorded on one-fourth standardization; 1 millivolt = 2.5 mm. Therefore, the R wave in V4 is 64 mm (16 × 4 = 64).

THE R/S RATIO

The measurement of the R/S ratio is important in the diagnosis of ventricular hypertrophy and is usually measured in V1, V2, and V6. The R/S ratio compares the amplitude of the R wave with that of the S wave.

In the example of Figure 1–10, the R/S ratio in V1 is 12 (18/1.5 = 12), and that in V2 is 1.8 (11/6 = 1.8). Although the calibration markers are one-half and one-fourth, respectively, the R/S ratio is not affected by the change in calibration factor.

THE QRS AXIS

What is the significance of the QRS axis? Since the QRS axis changes in disorders such as ventricular hypertrophy, bundle branch block, and other ventricular conduction disturbances, its calculation is helpful in the diagnosis of these conditions. The QRS axis that is routinely calculated in the scalar ECG is an approximation of the mean frontal plane vector of the QRS loop in the vectorcardiogram (VCG). One needs only the limb leads to calculate the QRS axis. A brief discussion of the VCG is presented later in this chapter.

Calculation may be made by the use of either a *graph* with triangular coordinates or the *hexaxial reference system*. The graph method is easy to learn but is inconvenient because one has to carry it at all times. The method using the hexaxial reference system requires memorization of the system but thereafter is more convenient to apply.

The Graph Method

Theoretically, one can use any two of the six limb leads for this purpose. In Figure 1–11,A leads I and III are used, and in Figure 1–11,B leads I and aVF are used.

Method

1. Find the net amplitude of the chosen two leads by subtracting the negative deflection from the positive deflection, and mark it on the appropriate limb of the axis of each lead.

2. Drop a perpendicular from each lead to find the intersection (*not* a parallelogram of forces).

3. Draw a line connecting the intersection and the center. This line is the QRS axis.

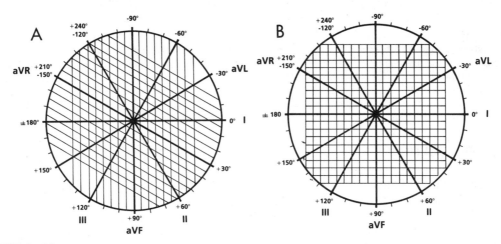

FIG 1–11.
Two graphs used in determining the QRS axis; both use two of the six limb leads. **A,** graph using leads I and III; **B,** graph using leads I and aVF.

Example (Fig 1–12)

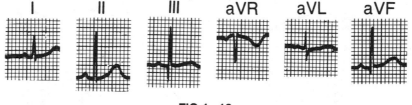

FIG 1–12.

Determine the QRS axis of Figure 1–12 using *Figure 1–11,A (leads I and III)*.

1. The net amplitude of lead I:
$$(+5.5) + (-0.5) = +5.0$$
(R wave = +5.5 mm, S wave = −0.5 mm)

2. The net amplitude of lead III:
$$(+10.0) + (-3.5) = +6.5$$
(R wave = +10 mm, Q wave = −3.5 mm)

3. Find the +5 point on lead I and +6.5 on lead III. (One may use any fraction or multiple of the numbers, if applied to both leads.) (Fig 1–13,A.)

4. Drop the perpendiculars from leads I and III to find the intersection.

5. The line connecting the intersection and the center of the circle defines the QRS axis. In this case it is +65 degrees (Fig 1–13,A).

Determine the QRS axis of Figure 1–12 using *Figure 1–11,B (leads I and aVF).*

1. The net amplitude of lead I = +5.0 (as above).

2. The net amplitude of aVF:
$$(+10.5) + (-1.5) = +9.0$$

3. Find the +5.0 point on lead I and the +9.0 point on aVF (Fig 1–13,B).

4. Connect the intersection of the perpendiculars with the center of the circle. The QRS axis is +60 degrees (Fig 1–13,B).

Note how close the two numbers are (+65 degrees and +60 degrees), although different figures were used.

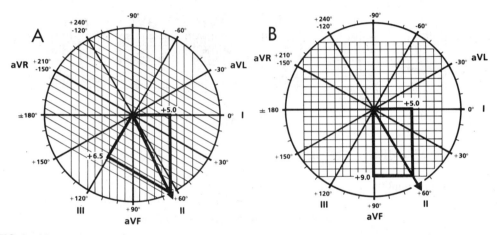

FIG 1–13.
Graph method using the two graphs shown in Figure 1–11. **A,** leads I and III are used. **B,** leads I and aVF are used.

Successive Approximation Method

It is necessary to memorize the hexaxial reference system (Fig 1–14). Leads I and aVF cross at right angles at the electrical center. The angle between any two adjacent leads is 30 degrees. The positive pole of each lead is indicated by the lead labels (Fig 1–14). The lead I axis represents the left-right relationship with the positive pole on the left and the negative pole on the right. The aVF lead represents the superior-inferior relationship with the positive pole directed inferiorly and the negative pole directed superiorly. The R wave in each lead represents the depolarization force directed toward the positive pole; the S wave, toward the negative pole. Therefore, the R wave of lead I represents the leftward force and the S wave of lead I the rightward force. By the same token, the R wave in aVF represents the inferiorly directed force and the S wave the superiorly directed force (Fig 1–15).

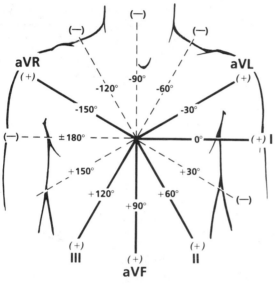

FIG 1–14.
Hexaxial reference system (viewed from the patient's front). Positive pole of each lead is indicated by (+) sign. The angle between two adjacent limb leads is 30 degrees.

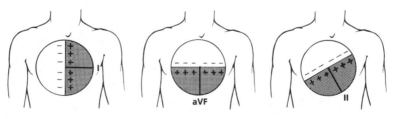

FIG 1–15.
Polarity of limb leads (viewed from the patient's front). Lines perpendicular to leads I, aVF, and III divide the areas into positive *(shaded)* and negative *(unshaded)* segments for polarity.

An easy way to memorize the system is shown in Figure 1–16 by a superimposition of a body with stretched arms and legs on the X and Y axes. The hands and feet are the positive poles or electrodes. The left and right hands are the positive poles of leads aVR and aVL, respectively. The left and right feet are the positive poles of leads II and III, respectively. The bipolar limb leads I, II, and III are clockwise in sequence for the positive electrode.

Method

Step 1: *Locate a quadrant, using leads I and aVF.* Depending on the deflections of the QRS complexes in leads I and aVF, the QRS axis may be in any one of the four quadrants (Fig 1–17). The way one locates the quadrant illustrated in the top panel of Figure 1–17 is explained step by step in Figure 1–18. The net QRS deflection is positive in lead I. This means that the QRS axis is in the left hemicircle (see Fig 1–18,A), which is the positive side of lead I (also see Fig 1–15). The net QRS complex is also positive in aVF, and this indicates that the axis is in the lower hemicircle (see Fig 1–18,B), the positive area from the lead aVF point of view. The QRS axis will be in the left lower quadrant (0 to +90 degrees) in order to satisfy the polarity of both leads I and aVF (see Fig 1–18,C).

Step 2a: *Find a lead with equiphasic QRS complex* (in which the height of R wave and the depth of S wave are equal). The QRS axis is perpendicular to the lead with equiphasic QRS complex, in the predetermined quadrant. Or:

Step 2b: *Find a lead with the greatest QRS deflection, either positive or negative, in the predetermined quadrant.* The QRS axis is close to the positive or negative limb of this lead.

FIG 1–16.
Easy way to memorize the hexaxial reference system (see text).

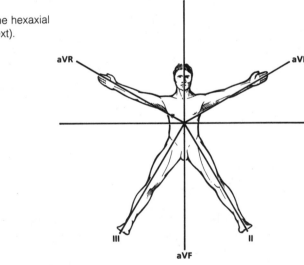

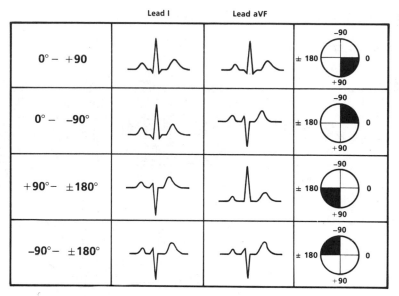

FIG 1–17.
Locating quadrants of mean QRS axis from leads I and aVF.

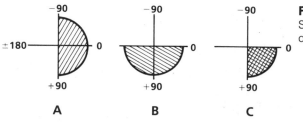

A   B   C

FIG 1–18.
Step-by-step method to determine a quadrant for mean QRS axis.

Three examples of QRS axis determination follow.

Example 1 (Fig 1–19,A)

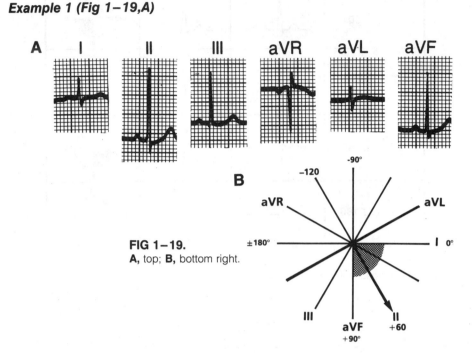

FIG 1–19.
A, top; **B,** bottom right.

Step 1: Using leads I and aVF, we find the QRS axis to be in the left lower quadrant (0 to 90 degrees) (Fig 1–19,B).

Step 2a: We find that the lead aVL has equiphasic QRS complexes. This means that the QRS axis is perpendicular to aVL, either +60 degrees or −120 degrees. Since we have already determined that the axis is in the 0 to +90 degree quadrant, the QRS axis is +60 rather than −120 degrees.

Step 2b: We find that the greatest deflection is the positive deflection of lead II. Therefore, the QRS axis is closest to lead II or +60 degrees.

Example 2 (Fig 1–20,A)

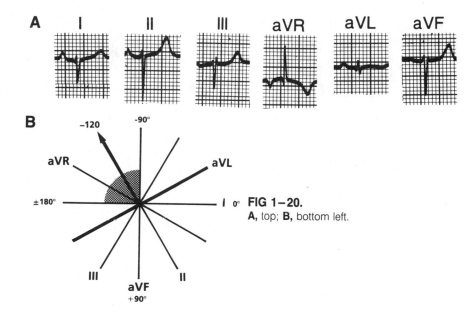

FIG 1–20.
A, top; **B,** bottom left.

Step 1: The QRS complexes are negative in lead I and negative in aVF, placing the axis in the right upper quadrant (−90 to −180 degrees) (Fig 1–20,B).

Step 2a: It is almost equiphasic in aVL, although slightly more positive. Therefore, the axis is close to −120 degrees.

Step 2b: Lead II has the deepest negative deflection. The negative limb of lead II is −120 degrees. The axis is *"indeterminate,"* that is, neither right nor left.

Example 3 (Fig 1–21,A)

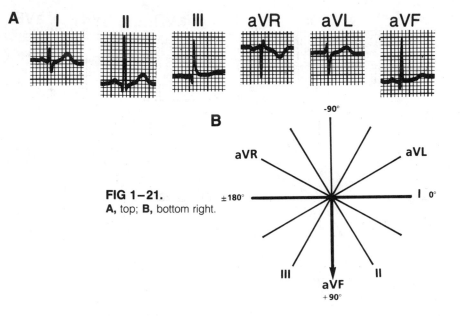

FIG 1–21.
A, top; **B,** bottom right.

Steps 1 and 2: The QRS complex is almost equiphasic in lead I. Therefore, the QRS axis is going to be either +90 or −90 degrees. Since the QRS is strongly positive in aVF, the axis is +90 degrees (Fig 1–21,B).

Two-Vector Plot

When the QRS complexes are equiphasic in many limb leads, as is seen in the Katz-Wachtel phenomenon (see Chap. 4, Hypertrophy), the QRS axis cannot be plotted in the usual manner just described. In this situation a more meaningful plot would consist of two vectors, one for the initial half *(initial QRS vector)* and one for the terminal half *(terminal QRS vector),* labeled QRSi and QRSt, respectively. This type of plot may also be useful when there are terminal slurrings (bundle branch block) and when there are Q waves equal to or greater than 0.03 second in duration (myocardial infarction). The graph method may be used to plot two vectors (see Figs 1–11,A or 1–11,B), although the method of successive approximation works equally well. Two examples of two-vector plot are presented.

Example 1 (Fig 1–22,A)

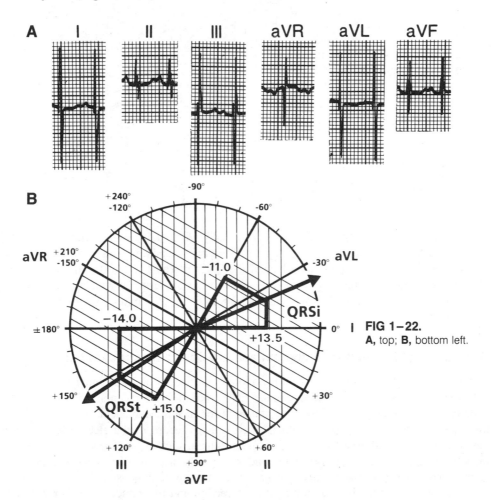

FIG 1–22.
A, top; **B,** bottom left.

 In Figure 1–22, there are large equiphasic QRS complexes in most of the limb leads. The initial portion of lead I consists of a small q (−1.5 mm) and a large R (+15 mm), with the net amplitude of +13.5 mm. The initial portion of lead III is made up by an r (+2.5 mm) and an S (−13.5 mm), with the net of −11 mm. Therefore, the QRSi is −20 degrees, using the method in Figure 1–11,A. The terminal QRS of lead I is −14 mm and that of lead III is +15 mm. Therefore, the QRSt is +145 degrees (Fig 1–22,B).

Example 2 (Fig 1–23,A)

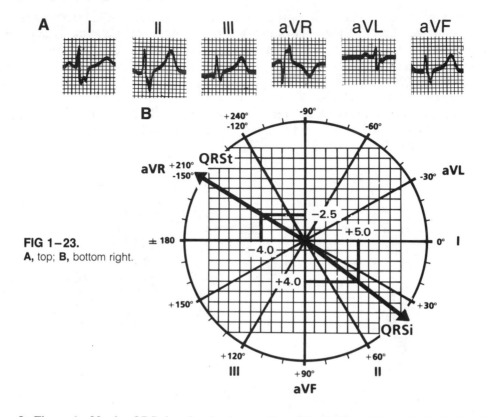

FIG 1–23.
A, top; **B,** bottom right.

In Figure 1–23, the QRS duration is abnormally wide (0.13), with terminal slurring (see Chap. 5), and the QRS complexes are equiphasic in many leads, making it difficult to plot the axis in the usual manner. The initial half of the QRS of lead I is +5.0 mm and that of lead aVF is +4.0 mm. Therefore, the QRSi is +40 degrees. The terminal wide portion of the QRS complex of lead I is −4.0 mm and that of lead aVF is −2.5 mm. Therefore, the QRSt is −150 degrees (Fig 1–23,B).

Correlation of the Vectorcardiogram and the Scalar Electrocardiogram

Although the vectorcardiogram (VCG) is no longer routinely obtained, understanding of VCG will help one understand the ordinary scalar ECG from the vectorial point of view. The VCG is defined as the registration of the time course of the mean instantaneous spatial cardiac vector. The VCG loop of the QRS complex is continuous record of the electromotive forces of the heart from two different scalar leads simultaneously, such as leads I and aVF. Records are made in three planes: frontal, horizontal, and sagittal. By inspecting two planes, especially the frontal and horizontal planes, one can gain important three-dimensional information of the electrical activity of the heart in terms of the direction and magnitude of the force as well as the direction of the inscription of the QRS loop. While the scalar ECG is more convenient when measuring intervals and amplitude, the VCG adds the important element of direction. The VCG and scalar ECG are two different ways of looking at the same electrical activity occurring in the heart. In fact, one can predict what the scalar ECG leads are going to look like from an assessment of the VCG (see subequent discussion).

A normal QRS loop in the frontal plane of a child is depicted in Figure 1–24. We will derive scalar ECGs from the VCG shown in this figure. In this exercise, we will consider three limb leads (I, II, and aVF), with detailed discussion of only lead I. The dotted line perpendicular to lead I indicates the isoelectric line for this lead. When looked at from the positive pole of lead I, it shows a small, initial negative vector (going away from the positive pole), producing a small q wave. The loop then makes a strong move toward the positive pole, crossing the baseline, which produces a large positive deflection (the upstroke of the R wave). This positive deflection then moves away from the positive electrode, producing the downstroke of the R wave, and then recrosses the isoelectric line, producing an S wave. In other words, any vector toward the subject's left (in the diagram to the right of the baseline) produces a positive deflection, and any vector to the left of the baseline produces a negative deflection.

By changing the position of the electrodes (or looking at the loop from different angles) and by using the same method, we can anticipate seeing a qRs pattern in lead II and a qR pattern in aVF as shown in Figure 1–24.

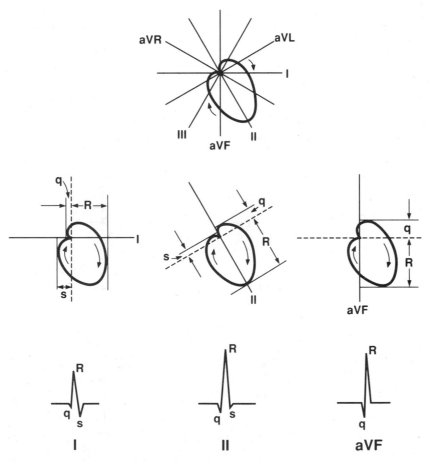

FIG 1–24.
Frontal plane QRS loop commonly seen in normal children. There is a clockwise loop with the maximal QRS vector toward +60 degrees.

Normal Vectorcardiographic QRS Loop

The normal vectorcardiographic QRS loop of the newborn and the adult is different in terms of orientation and/or the direction of inscription of the loop (Fig 1–25). In the *frontal plane* of the VCG of normal newborns, the major vector is to the subject's right and inferior, and the direction of inscription of the QRS loop is clockwise. This is reflective of the fact that the RV is the dominant ventricle at this age. In older children and adults, the major QRS vector is to the left and inferior, while maintaining the clockwise loop in the majority of normal subjects. In some adults, the direction of inscription is counterclockwise. Therefore, as a newborn infant grows up, there is a gradual leftward shift of the QRS vector from the right lower quadrant to the left lower quadrant, without changes in the direction of inscription. In the scalar ECG, this change is expressed as a gradual change in the QRS axis from the right lower quadrant to the left lower quadrant. This change in the QRS vector reflects the progression from RV dominance in the newborn to LV dominance in the adult.

In the *horizontal plane,* the QRS loop of the newborn is in the right and anterior quadrant (reflecting the RV dominance of this age), with the direction of inscription clockwise. In the adult, the QRS loop is in the left posterior quadrant (reflecting normal LV dominance), with the direction of the loop counterclockwise (see Fig 1–25). In order for a clockwise loop in the right-anterior quadrant seen in the newborn to change to a counterclockwise loop in the left-posterior quadrant seen in the adult, somewhat complex changes must take place in the horizontal plane. A detailed discussion of this aspect will be presented later in Chapter 5, Ventricular Conduction Disturbances. At that time, the reasons for unusual rsR′ patterns and notched R or S waves seen in V1 of infants' ECGs will be discussed.

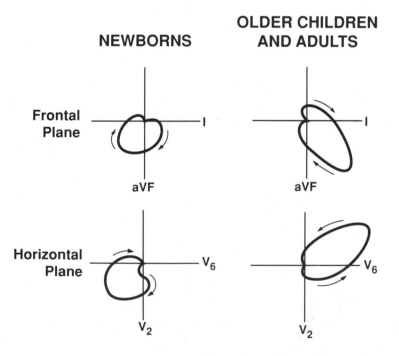

FIG 1–25.

Comparison of vectorcardiographic QRS loops in the frontal and horizontal planes of normal newborn infants and adults (see text). The *arrows* indicate the direction of inscription of the loops.

THE P AXIS AND T AXIS

The same methods used to determine the QRS axis can be used for the P axis and T axis, the only difference being that one looks for a lead with flat P and T waves if equiphasic waves are not found.

P Axis

What is the significance of the P axis? The P axis represents the direction of the atrial depolarization vector and therefore gives information about the pacemaker site and the location of the sinoatrial (SA) node. Accordingly, it is important in the interpretation of abnormal rhythm and chamber localization (see Chaps. 7 and 8). Two examples of P-axis determination follow (Figs 1–26 and 1–27).

Example 1 (Fig 1–26)

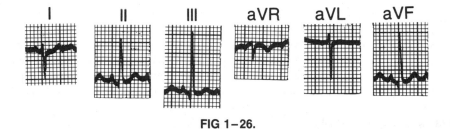

FIG 1–26.

   In Figure 1–26, since the P waves are positive in leads I and aVF, the P axis is in the left lower quadrant (0 to +90 degrees). In most instances that is enough evidence to say there is *sinus rhythm:* i.e., the SA node is the pacemaker (see Chap. 7, arrhythmias). (In sinus rhythm, the P axis is directed anteriorly as well. This is shown as a positive P wave in V1 and V2). To be more precise, we find a flat P wave in aVL; therefore, it is perpendicular to aVL and the P axis is +60 degrees.

Example 2 (Fig 1–27)

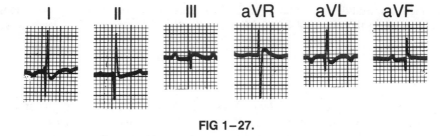

FIG 1–27.

In Figure 1–27, the negative P in lead I and the positive P in aVF place the P axis in the right lower quadrant (+90 to +180 degrees). The P is almost flat (although slightly positive) in aVR. Therefore, the P axis is +120 degrees or slightly greater. This is an abnormal P axis. This patient has mirror-image dextrocardia (see Chap. 8).

T Axis

The T axis represents the mean vector of ventricular repolarization. It is important because it changes in major disorders such as severe ventricular hypertrophy (with "strain"), ventricular conduction disturbances, and other myocardial disorders. A full discussion will be presented in chapters 4, 5, and 6. Two examples of T axis determination follow (Figs 1–28 and 1–29).

Example 1 (Fig 1–28)

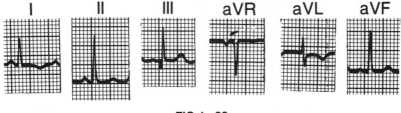

FIG 1–28.

In Figure 1–28, the negative T in lead I and the positive T in aVF place the T axis in the right lower quadrant (+90 to +180 degrees). The T wave is flat in aVR, and therefore the T axis is close to lead III (+120 degrees). In fact, the T waves are the tallest in lead III, confirming the T axis of +120 degrees.

Example 2 (Fig 1–29)

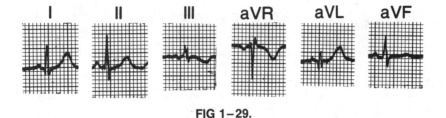

FIG 1–29.

In Figure 1–29, the T waves are upright in leads I and aVF. Therefore, the T axis is in the 0 to +90 degree-quadrant. The T wave is the tallest in lead I and the smallest in aVF. This means that the T axis is close to 0 degrees but still more than 0 degrees (because of the upright T in aVF), or about +10 degrees.

THE QRS-T ANGLE

Since the QRS-T angle relates the depolarization activity to the ventricular repolarization, it is important in the diagnosis of severe ventricular hypertrophy (with "strain"), ventricular conduction disturbances, and other repolarization abnormalities of the ventricle. The QRS-T angle is simply the angle formed by the QRS axis and the T axis. Two examples are given in Figures 1–34 and 1–35.

HORIZONTAL REFERENCE SYSTEM

The QRS axis we have discussed so far relates to the frontal plane of the vectorcardiogram (VCG). In other words, the QRS axis determined from the hexaxial reference system tells us the left-right and the superior-inferior relationships but does not give information about the

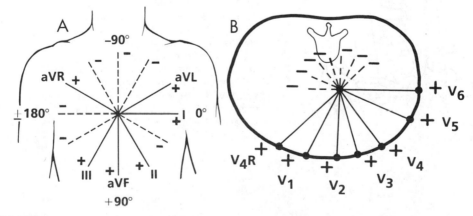

FIG 1–30.
Hexaxial **(A)** and horizontal **(B)** reference systems. (Hexaxial reference system is shown again for comparison.)

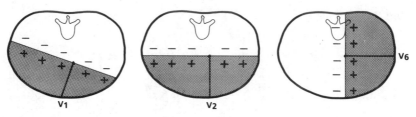

FIG 1–31.
Polarity of precordial leads. Lines drawn perpendicular to leads V1, V2, and V6 divide the areas into positive *(shaded)* and negative *(unshaded)* segments for polarity.

anterior-posterior relationship. Information about the anterior-posterior and the left-right relationship, which is gained from the horizontal plane of the VCG, can be constructed from the precordial leads using the horizontal reference system.

The horizontal reference system is not as precise as the hexaxial reference system (Fig 1–30,A), in which the angle between the two adjacent leads is 30 degrees. The approximate relationship of the precordial leads is illustrated in Figure 1–30,B. The positive pole of each lead is indicated by the lead labels (V4R, V1, V2, etc.). The leads V2 and V6 cross at a right angle at the electrical center of the heart. The V6 axis represents the left-right relationship with the positive pole on the left and the negative pole on the right. The V2 axis represents the anterior-posterior relationship with the positive pole anterior and the negative pole posterior. Therefore, the R wave in V6 represents the leftward forces and the R wave of V2 the anterior forces. Conversely, the S wave in V6 represents the rightward forces and the S wave of V2 the posterior forces. The R wave in V1 represents the anterior *and* rightward forces and the S wave the posterior and leftward forces (Fig 1–31). Although the S in V2 usually represents posterior or left ventricular forces, in the presence of marked right axis deviation the S in V2 may represent right ventricular force that is directed rightward and posteriorly (see Figs 9–13 and 9–16).

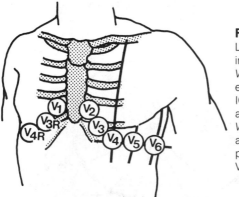

FIG 1–32.
Location of precordial leads: *V1,* fourth intercostal space (ICS) at the right sternal border; *V2,* fourth ICS at the left sternal border; *V3,* equidistant point between V2 and V4; *V4,* fifth ICS in the left midclavicular line; *V5,* anterior axillary line in the same horizontal plane as V4; *V6,* midaxillary line in the same horizontal plane as V4. V3R, V4R, V5R, and V6R are mirror image points (on the right side of the chest) of V3, V4, V5, and V6, respectively.

So far we have discussed only the theoretical aspects of the horizontal reference system. Figure 1–32 illustrates the position for the actual placement of the precordial leads. Placing the electrodes one space higher or lower results in precordial leads that are quite different from those placed at the right level. An example of misplacing the electrodes is shown in Figure A–2 (Appendix).

The anterior-posterior relationship may be incorporated into the hexaxial reference system by the use of an arrow. The V2 lead is the best lead to determine whether the vector of the QRS complex, the T wave or the P wave, is anterior or posterior. Figure 1–33 illustrates how one determines whether the QRS vector is anterior or posterior and how to draw it using an arrow. If the QRS complex is predominantly positive (or upright), the vector is anterior; and if the QRS is predominantly negative (or downward), the vector is posterior. The same method is used for determination of the P or T vector.

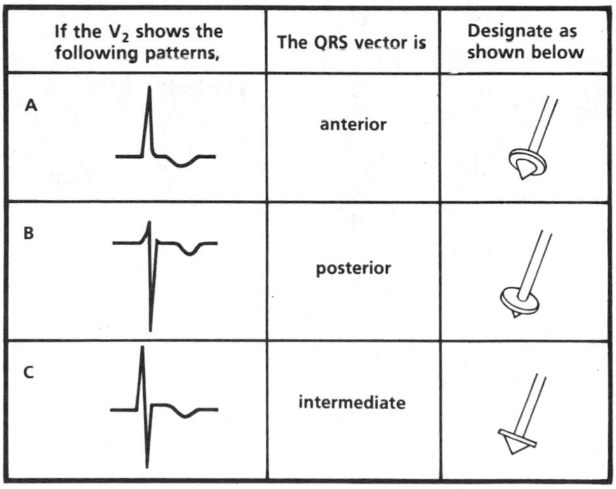

If the V₂ shows the following patterns,	The QRS vector is	Designate as shown below
A	anterior	
B	posterior	
C	intermediate	

FIG 1–33.
A method to show anterior or posterior QRS vector in the horizontal plane. The T vector is posterior in each plane. Right axis deviation was present in the limb leads, not shown here.

The following two examples (Figs 1–34 and 1–35) show how to draw the QRS axis and the T axis with their anterior or posterior directions shown, and how to determine the QRS-T angle.

Example 1 (Fig 1–34,A)

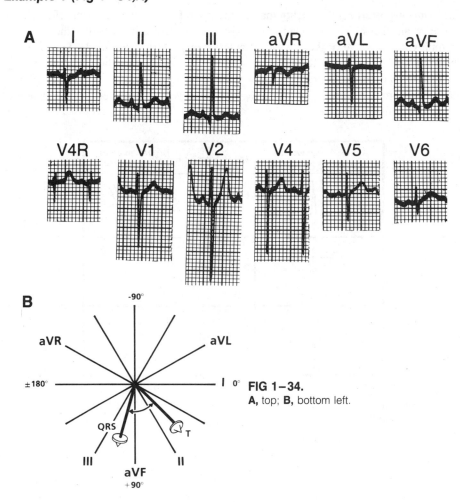

FIG 1–34.
A, top; **B,** bottom left.

The QRS axis in the frontal plane (on the hexaxial system) is +105 degrees. The QRS vector must be posterior since there is a deep S in V2. Therefore, the arrow is drawn as pointing posteriorly (Fig 1–34,B). The T axis is +45 degrees, and the arrow points anteriorly. The QRS-T angle is 60 degrees.

Example 2 (Fig 1–35,A)

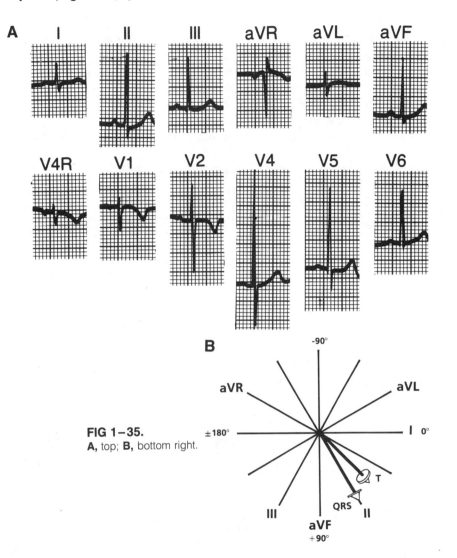

FIG 1–35.
A, top; **B,** bottom right.

In Figure 1–35, the QRS axis on the hexaxial system is +60 degrees. The QRS is equal in the anterior and posterior directions (intermediate). Therefore, we draw the arrow as in Figure 1–35,B. The T axis is +45 degrees, pointing posteriorly. Therefore, the QRS-T angle is 15 degrees.

MORPHOLOGY OF ECG DEFLECTIONS

The QRS Complex

The initial negative (downward) deflection is called a Q wave and the initial positive (upward) deflection an R wave. A negative deflection after the R wave is called an S wave. A secondary positive deflection after the S wave is labeled R′ and a secondary negative wave after the R′ is called S′. When there is only a negative deflection (without discernible R) in the QRS complex, it is called a QS complex. Capital letters are used to describe the major deflection or a deflection that is at least one half the amplitude of the major deflection. Lower-case letters are used to describe minor deflections with less than one half the amplitude of the major deflection.

Examples of common QRS wave forms are shown in Figure 1–36.

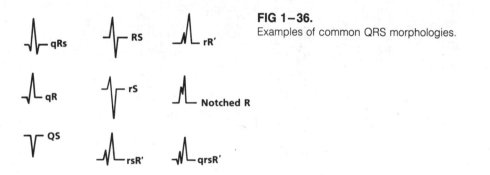

FIG 1–36.
Examples of common QRS morphologies.

The P and T Waves and ST Segments

Common forms of P and T waves and ST segments are presented in Figure 1–37.

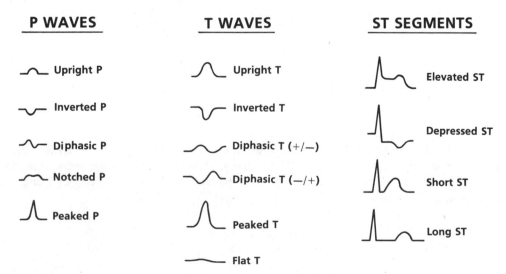

FIG 1–37.
Common morphologies of the P wave, T wave, and ST segment.

REVIEW QUESTIONS

1. Calculate the heart rate in each of the examples in Figure 1–38.

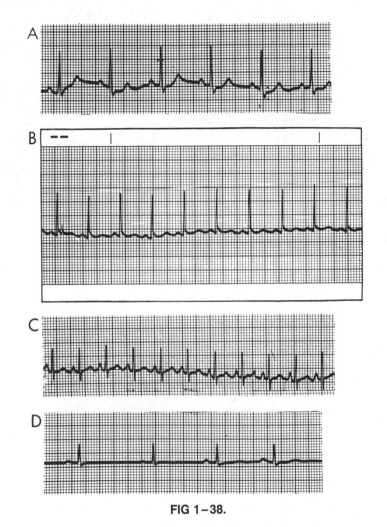

FIG 1–38.

2. Which of the following QRS deflections does *not* represent rightward force?
   a. R in aVR
   b. S in I
   c. R in II
   d. S in aVL

3. A positive QRS complex in lead I and a negative QRS in aVF place the QRS axis in which of the following quadrants?
   a. 0 to +90 degrees
   b. +90 to +180 degrees
   c. 0 to −90 degrees
   d. −90 to −180 degrees

4. Plot the P, QRS, and T axes of the ECG in Figure 1–39 and determine the QRS-T angle.

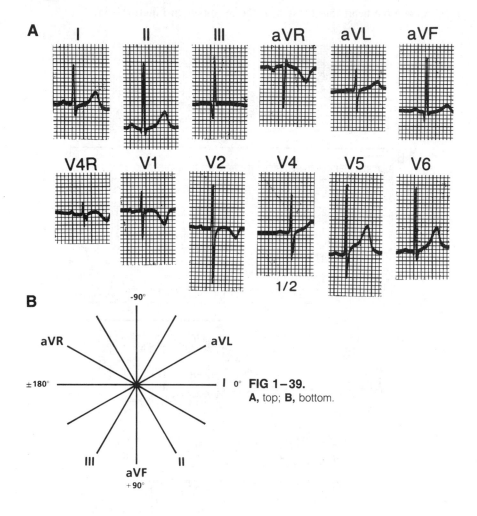

FIG 1–39.
A, top; **B,** bottom.

5. Is the QRS vector anterior, posterior, or intermediate in the tracing in Figure 1–39?
6. All but one of the following statements are correct; which is incorrect?
   a. The Q wave represents atrial depolarization.
   b. The conduction velocity through the AV node is slower than that through the atrial myocardium.
   c. The T wave represents ventricular repolarization.
   d. The QRS complex represents ventricular depolarization.

7. Determine the initial and terminal QRS vectors of the ECG in Figure 1–40.

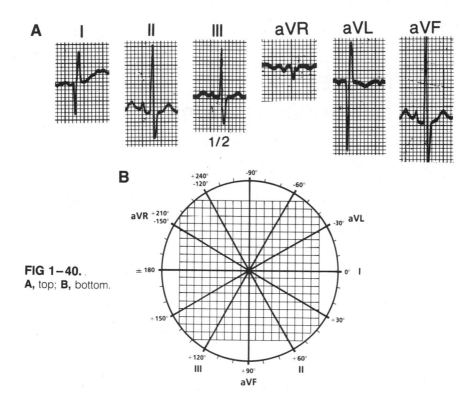

FIG 1–40.
A, top; **B,** bottom.

Answer the following questions either "true" or "false."

8. The R wave in lead I represents leftward force.	True	False
9. The S wave in aVF represents the superiorly directed force.	True	False
10. An equiphasic QRS complex in aVL and a predominant R wave in lead II place the QRS axis at +60 degrees.	True	False
11. P waves positive in leads II and aVF indicate sinus rhythm.	True	False
12. The S wave in V1 represents rightward and posterior force.	True	False
13. The R wave in V2 represents leftward force.	True	False
14. The PR interval is measured from the onset of the P wave to the peak of the R wave.	True	False
15. With one-half standardization, 10 mm deflection should be read as 5 mm.	True	False

Answers may be found on page 238.

CHAPTER 2

Normal Electrocardiograms

In this chapter anatomical reasons are presented for the differences in the electrocardiograms (ECGs) of newborns compared with older children. The differences between the ECGs of premature and full-term newborn infants are also discussed. Typical ECG tracings of children of various ages are shown, with a description of the important features.

AGE-RELATED CHANGES IN ECG

Most of the age-related changes in pediatric ECGs are related to the changes in the ratio of left ventricular (LV) to right ventricular (RV) weight. At birth the right ventricle (RV) is thicker than the left ventricle (LV). There is such a large increase in LV weight during the first month that by the end of that month the LV is heavier than the RV. The ratio of LV/RV reaches about 2:1 by 6 months of age. Thereafter, the ratio increases very slowly to a value of about 2.5:1 by the time of young adulthood (Table 2–1).

The ECG reflects this anatomical change. The normal RV dominance of the newborn period is gradually replaced by the LV dominance of later childhood and adulthood. The ECG changes are more rapid in the first month of life than afterward, as can be expected from the anatomical changes. There is a tremendous variation of the norm at each age group, but in general the younger the age group the wider is the range of normal.

The following general changes occur with increasing age:

1. The heart rate decreases.
2. All the durations and intervals (PR interval, QRS duration, QT interval) increase.

TABLE 2–1.
LV/RV Weight Ratio

30 weeks gestation	1.2:1
33 weeks gestation	1.0:1
36 weeks gestation	0.8:1
At birth	0.8:1
1 month	1.5:1
6 months	2.0:1
Adult	2.5:1

3. RV dominance in the infant gradually changes to LV dominance in the adult.
   a. The QRS axis changes from the right and anterior direction in infants, to the left and posterior direction in adults.
   b. The R wave amplitude in the right precordial leads (RPL) decreases, and in the left precordial leads (LPL) it increases.
   c. The S wave voltage in the RPL increases, and in the LPL it decreases.
   d. The R/S ratio in the RPL decreases, and in the LPL it increases.
4. The marked anteriorness of the T vector in newborn infants disappears within a few days. During childhood, it remains intermediate. Beginning at 8 to 10 years, the T vector gradually moves anteriorly.

ECG of Premature Infants

There is a slight but definite difference in the ECG of premature infants compared with that of full-term newborn infants as a group. This is partly due to the difference in the relative weight of the ventricles in that premature infants have less right ventricular dominance (or more left ventricular dominance) than full-term infants. The LV/RV ratio is about 1.2:1 at 30 weeks gestation, 1:1 at 33 weeks gestation, and 0.8:1 at 36 weeks gestation (see Table 2–1).

In comparison to the full-term infant, the ECG of the premature infant shows the following:

1. Lower voltages of the QRS complex and T wave in the standard limb leads.
2. Less RV dominance and more leftward forces:
   a. T waves in V1 are almost invariably negative (less RV dominance). (T waves are commonly upright in V1 in full-term infants, suggesting more right dominance.)
   b. There is a higher incidence of deep Q in V6 and more leftward QRS axis (LV dominance).

A study comparing premature and mature infants of similar weight also reveals:

1. A tendency toward relative LV dominance for the premature group (QRS axis more to the left, taller R in V6, smaller R in V4R and V1, and taller T in V6).
2. Relatively shorter PR, QRS, and QT intervals in the premature group.
3. More variability in the ECG of the premature infant than in that of the full-term infant.

Although there is a difference between premature and full-term newborn infants, there is so much overlap in the range of normal between the two groups that the normal data for full-term infants can be used for evaluating premature infants (see Chap. 3). Normal data for premature infants are presented here for the sake of completeness (Table 2–2).

NORMAL ECG TRACINGS

A general description of the normal ECG is presented with a representative tracing for different age groups. Details of each description are intended to emphasize changes in ECG patterns with increasing age. The ECGs of newborns and infants younger than 1 month normally show right axis deviation (RAD) and right ventricular dominance. Children 3 years of age and older should have an ECG that resembles an adult ECG. Between 1 month and 3 years of age, ECGs are intermediate, showing neither right nor left ventricular dominance. It is in this age group that many normal ECGs show large QRS deflections in the precordial leads, findings suggestive of combined ventricular hypertrophy (CVH).

TABLE 2–2.
R and S Voltages in Premature Infants*†‡

Leads	R Voltages, Mean (Upper Limits)		S Voltages, Mean (Upper Limits)	
	1–7 days	1 wk–1 mo	1–7 days	1 wk–1 mo
I	2 (6)	3 (9)	3 (10)	3 (6)
II	6 (13)	7 (15)		
III	7 (14)	8 (16)		
aVR	3 (8)	2 (4)		
aVL	2 (4)	2 (6)		
aVF	7 (16)	9 (16)		
V4R	11 (21)	7 (17)		
V2	15 (27)	14 (25)	14 (28)	13 (25)
V6	7 (15)	10 (17)	7 (22)	5 (13)

*Voltages are in mm deflection.
†Weight of premature infants, 1,000 to 2,500 gm.
‡Modified from Levin OR, Griffiths SP: *Pediatrics* 1962; 30:361–371.

Newborn (Fig 2–1)

1. Relatively small QRS voltages in the limb leads.
2. Right axis deviation (up to +180 degrees).
3. The precordial leads show right ventricular dominance:
   a. Tall R waves in the RPLs, but pure R in V1 is rare. (Pure R in V1 of more than 10 mm is strongly suggestive of right ventricular hypertrophy).
   b. Deep S waves in the LPLs (V5 and V6).
   c. R/S ratio is greater than 1 in the RPLs and is relatively small in the LPLs.
   d. Complete reversal of adult R/S progression (see Fig 2–7) is common.
4. The T waves are of low voltages.
5. The T wave in V1 may be upright in an infant on the first day of life, but it usually becomes negative by 3 days of age; if not, RVH is suggested.
6. A q wave in V4R with a qRS pattern is uncommon but is not necessarily abnormal as long as there is a q wave in V6. (Careful inspection of V4R may reveal an rsR'S' pattern.) A qR pattern in V1 is very unusual and is suggestive of RVH, although the same caution relative to small initial r waves is required.

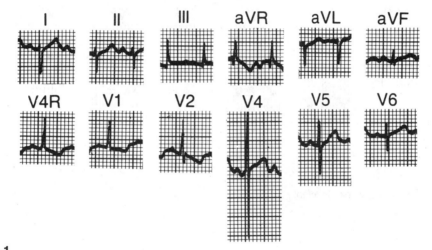

FIG 2–1.
ECG from a normal newborn infant.

1 Week – 1 Month (Fig 2–2)

1. Retains right axis deviation (see Fig 3–2).
2. Still has a dominant R wave in the RPLs.
3. The R wave is dominant in V6, although if a dominant S is found, it is within the normal limits.
4. The T waves in the limb leads are of higher voltages than in newborn infants.
5. The T waves in V1 are almost always negative. (Upright T in V1 in infants older than 3 days of age is suggestive of RVH.)
6. Adult type R/S progression in the precordial leads (see Fig 2–7) is rarely seen in the first month of life. (If it is present, left ventricular hypertrophy should be suspected.)

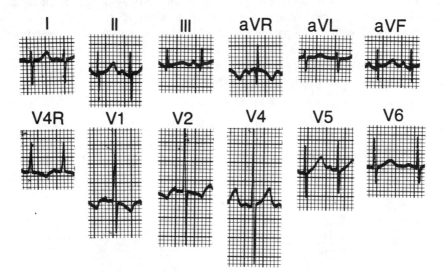

FIG 2–2.
ECG from a normal 2-week-old infant.

1—6 Months (Fig 2—3)

1. Reduction of the rightward QRS axis. The QRS axis is usually less than +90 degrees, but up to +125 degrees is considered normal (see Fig 3—2).
2. The R/S ratio in V2 is close to 1, but the mean ratio in V1 is still greater than 1.
3. The R wave continues to be dominant in V4R and V1.
4. The T wave in V1 remains negative.
5. RSR′ pattern in V1 is not abnormal for this age group, provided that the QRS duration and amplitude are not abnormal (see Chap. 5, Ventricular Conduction Disturbances, for further discussion).
6. Many ECGs in children of this age are suggestive of combined ventricular hypertrophy (CVH) because of large QRS deflections in the precordial leads.

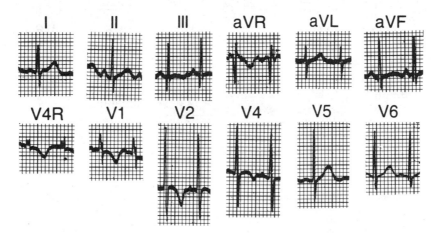

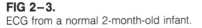

FIG 2—3.
ECG from a normal 2-month-old infant.

6 Months–3 Years (Fig 2–4)

1. The QRS axis is usually less than +90 degrees.
2. The R/S ratio in V1 becomes close to or less than 1.
3. The R wave is clearly dominant in V6.
4. Again, many children of this age have ECG findings compatible with CVH because of large QRS deflections in the precordial leads.

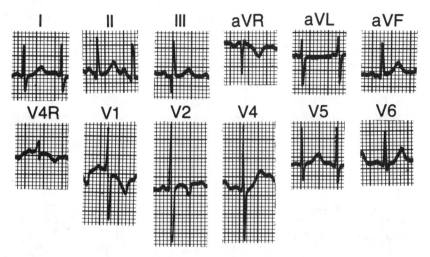

FIG 2–4.
ECG from a normal 14-month-old infant.

3–8 Years (Fig 2–5)

1. The adult R/S progression in the precordial leads is the rule (dominant S in the RPLs and dominant R waves in the LPLs).
2. Relatively large potentials are still seen in the RPLs.
3. The Q waves in the LPLs are of relatively large amplitude but are usually less than 5 mm.

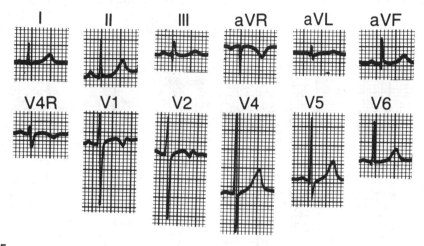

FIG 2–5.
ECG from a normal 5-year-old child.

8–16 Years (Fig 2–6)

1. The QRS axis is 0 to +90 degrees, with a mean of +60 degrees.
2. The adult QRS pattern or adult R/S progression is seen (dominant S in the RPLs and dominant R in the LPLs).
3. Relatively large amplitude of the QRS complex in the precordial leads. The R waves in the LPLs are greater than those in the adult.
4. The T waves in V1 may be upright. Negative T waves are *not* abnormal in V1 to V4.

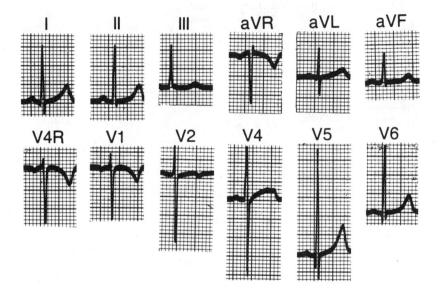

FIG 2–6.
ECG from a normal 12-year-old child.

Adults (Fig 2–7)

1. The QRS axis is 0 to +100 degrees, with a mean of +50 degrees.
2. The left ventricle is dominant (dominant S in the RPLs and dominant R in the LPLs, the *adult R/S progression*).
3. The T waves are usually anteriorly oriented (upright T in V2 through V6, and even in V1).
4. The PR interval is less than 0.20. The QRS duration is less than 0.10.

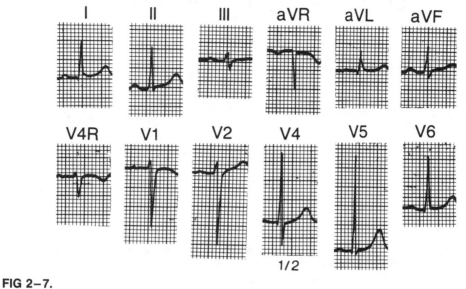

FIG 2–7.
ECG from a normal young adult.

REVIEW QUESTIONS

Answer the following questions either "true" or "false."

1. At birth the right ventricle is thicker than the left ventricle.	True	False
2. The dominant QRS deflection of V1 is an S in a newborn infant.	True	False
3. The R/S ratio in V2 is less than 1 in normal adults.	True	False
4. Premature infants have relatively more right ventricular dominance than full-term newborn infants.	True	False
5. The T waves are upright in V1 throughout childhood and adulthood.	True	False
6. The amplitude of R waves is usually greater than that of the S waves in the right precordial leads in a newborn infant less than 1 month of age.	True	False
7. In 6-month-old infants, the R/S ratio in V2 is close to 1.	True	False
8. By the time a child is 3 to 8 years of age, precordial leads will assume the adult QRS pattern, i.e., dominant S in V1 and dominant R in V6.	True	False
9. The mean adult QRS axis is +50 degrees.	True	False

Answers may be found on page 238.

CHAPTER 3

Normal ECG Values and Deviations From Normal

In this chapter normal electrocardiographic values in children are presented according to age and are followed by a list of conditions with abnormal values. Memorization is not required, but access to these tables is necessary for accurate interpretation of the electrocardiogram (ECG) in the pediatric age group.

HEART RATE

The heart rate of pediatric patients varies with age, status at the time of ECG recording (awake, sleeping, crying), as well as other physical factors such as fever. Normal heart rates according to age are as follows:

Newborn	110–150
2 years	85–125
4 years	75–115
6 years	65–100
Older than 6 years	60–100

Because of this age-related variation, the definitions used for adults of bradycardia (less than 60) or tachycardia (in excess of 100) are not helpful in discriminating normal from abnormal in pediatric patients. Operationally, *tachycardia* is present when the heart rate is faster than the ranges of normal for that age. Tachycardia may be caused by one of the following:

1. Sinus tachycardia.
2. Supraventricular tachycardia (atrial, nodal/AV junctional, or reentry).
3. Ventricular tachycardia.
4. Atrial fibrillation.
5. Atrial flutter.

Bradycardia is present when the heart rate is slower than the lower range of normal for that age, and it may be due to:

1. Sinus bradycardia.
2. Nodal rhythm.
3. Second-degree atrioventricular block (AV block).
4. Third-degree (complete) AV block.

RHYTHM

The normal rhythm for any age is sinus rhythm, in which the sinoatrial (SA) node is the pace-maker of the entire heart. There must be a P wave (only one) in front of each QRS complex, and the P axis must be in the range of 0 to +90 degrees. Therefore, P waves are upright in lead II and usually upright in leads I and aVF.

Abnormal, or nonsinus, rhythm is suggested by the presence of either abnormal number or shape of the P waves or abnormal P axis.

Abnormal Rhythm

1. The *absence of P waves* indicates a nonsinus rhythm (abnormalities in the impulse formation) and is seen in:
   a. Sinoatrial block (SA block).
   b. AV junctional (or nodal) rhythm.
   c. Atrial fibrillation.
   d. Idioventricular rhythm.
2. *Multiple P waves* (per QRS complex) are seen in:
   a. Atrial flutter.
   b. Atrial fibrillation.
   c. Atrial tachycardia with block.
   d. AV block, second or third degree.
3. *Changing P wave shape* is an indication of:
   a. Wandering atrial pacemaker.
4. *Abnormal P axis* (see below for discussion).
   a. Atrial inversion (situs inversus).
   b. Retrograde activation from AV node.
   c. Ectopic atrial pacemaker.

P WAVE

P Axis

The P axis represents the direction of the atrial depolarization vector. Therefore, it gives information about the pacemaker site: whether it is the sinoatrial (SA) node, atria, or the AV junctional (nodal) region. The normal P axis ranges from 0 to +90 degrees at any age.

Abnormal P Axis

1. A P axis in the right lower quadrant (or more than +90 degrees) is seen in:
   a. Atrial inversion.
   b. Incorrectly placed arm leads.
2. A superiorly oriented P axis (P axis less than 0 degrees) may be seen in (see Chap. 7, Arrhythmias):
   a. Nodal (or AV junctional) rhythm with retrograde conduction.
   b. Low ectopic atrial pacemaker ("coronary sinus" rhythm).

P Amplitude

The mean P amplitude in lead II or any other lead is about 1.5 mm with a maximum of 3.0 mm. Tall P waves (greater than 3 mm) are an indication of right atrial hypertrophy (RAH or "p-pulmonale") (see Chap. 4, Hypertrophy).

P Duration

The P wave duration is the time required for the depolarization of the atria (Fig 3–1). Normal average P wave duration is 0.06 ± 0.02 second in children. The maximal P duration is 0.10 second in normal children and 0.08 second in infants less than 12 months of age.

Prolongation of P wave duration (wide and often notched) is seen in left atrial hypertrophy (LAH or "p-mitrale") (see Chap. 4, Hypertrophy).

PR INTERVAL

PR interval is the time required for atrial depolarization (P duration) and the physiologic delay of the impulse in the AV node (PQ segment) (see Fig 3–1). The normal PR interval varies with *age* and *heart rate*. The older the person and the slower the heart rate, the longer is the PR interval. The mean and upper limits of normal (ULN) PR interval according to age and

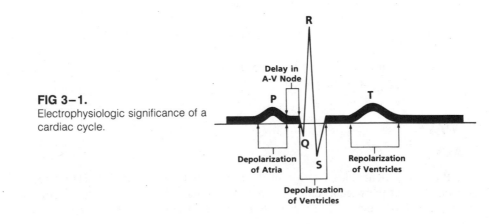

FIG 3–1.
Electrophysiologic significance of a cardiac cycle.

TABLE 3–1.

PQ (PR) Interval, With Rate and Age (and Upper Limits of Normal)

Rate	0–1 mo	1–6 mo	6 mo–1 yr	1–3 yr	3–8 yr	8–12 yr	12–16 yr	Adult
<60						0.16(0.18)	0.16(0.19)	0.17(0.21)
60–80					0.15(0.17)	0.15(0.17)	0.15(0.18)	0.16(0.21)
80–100	0.10(0.12)				0.14(0.16)	0.15(0.16)	0.15(0.17)	0.15(0.20)
100–120	0.10(0.12)			(0.15)	0.13(0.16)	0.14(0.15)	0.15(0.16)	0.15(0.19)
120–140	0.10(0.11)	0.11(0.14)	0.11(0.14)	0.12(0.14)	0.13(0.15)	0.14(0.15)		0.15(0.18)
140–160	0.09(0.11)	0.10(0.13)	0.11(0.13)	0.11(0.14)	0.12(0.14)			(0.17)
160–180	0.10(0.11)	0.10(0.12)	0.10(0.12)	0.10(0.12)				
>180	0.09	0.09(0.11)	0.10(0.11)					

Modified from Guntheroth WG: *Pediatric Electrocardiography*. Philadelphia, WB Saunders Co, 1965.

heart rate are presented in Table 3–1. The lower limits of normal PR interval according to age are as follows:

Less than 3 years	0.08 second
3 to 16 years	0.10 second
More than 16 years	0.12 second

Abnormal PR Interval

1. *Prolongation of PR interval* (first-degree AV block) usually indicates an abnormal delay in the conduction through the AV node and may be seen in:
   a. Myocarditis; rheumatic, viral, or diphtheric.
   b. Certain congenital heart defects (endocardial cushion defect, atrial septal defect [ASD], Ebstein's anomaly).
   c. Toxicity; digitalis, quinidine, etc.
   d. Hyperkalemia.
   e. Ischemia or profound hypoxia.
   f. Otherwise normal heart.
2. *Short PR interval* may be seen in:
   a. Wolff-Parkinson-White syndrome (WPW syndrome).
   b. Lown-Ganong-Levine syndrome.
   c. Glycogen storage disease.
3. *Variable PR intervals* are seen in:
   a. Wandering atrial pacemaker.
   b. Wenckebach phenomenon (Mobitz type I second-degree AV block).

QRS COMPLEX

QRS Axis

The QRS axis represents the mean vector of the ventricular depolarization process. The newborn infant normally has right axis deviation (RAD) compared to the adult standard. The mean QRS axis is +125 degrees, but up to +180 degrees is considered normal in the newborn period. The mean QRS axis of +90 degrees is reached by the time the child is 1 month of age and there is a gradual change to the left throughout childhood, approaching the adult mean value of +50 degrees by 3 years of age. However, the range for normal persons is wide (Fig 3–2 shows its normal range). The mean QRS axis according to age is as follows:

Newborn	+125 degrees
1 month	+90 degrees
3 years	+60 degrees
Adult	+50 degrees

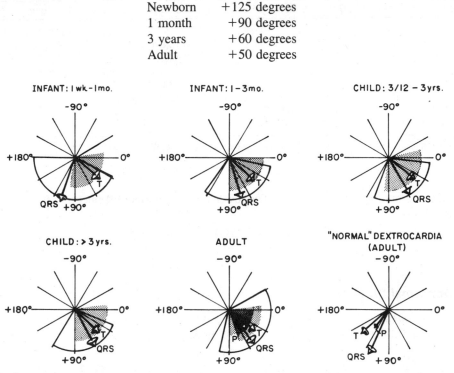

FIG 3–2.
Normal ranges for QRS and T axes according to age of the child. Normal range of P axis is also shown for the adult. "Normal" dextrocardia is synonymous with "mirror-image" dextrocardia. *Shaded area* is the normal range of T axis, *unshaded, fan-shaped area* is the normal range of QRS axis. Mean of each is shown by *arrows* and *labels*. (From Guntheroth WG: *Pediatric Electrocardiography*. Philadelphia, WB Saunders Co, 1965. Used by permission.)

Abnormal QRS Axis

Figure 3–3 shows the typical abnormal QRS and T axes in ventricular hypertrophy and conduction disturbances.

1. *Left axis deviation (LAD)* is present when the QRS axis is less than the lower limit of normal for that age. It occurs with:
    a. Left ventricular hypertrophy (LVH), particularly with volume overload lesions.
    b. Left bundle branch block (LBBB).
    c. Left anterior hemiblock.
2. *Right axis deviation (RAD)* is present when the QRS axis is greater than the upper limit of normal for age. It occurs with:
    a. Right ventricular hypertrophy (RVH).
    b. Right bundle branch block (RBBB).

3. Superiorly oriented axis *(superior axis)* is present when the S wave is greater than the R wave in aVF (note overlap with LAD). It may occur with:
   a. Left anterior hemiblock, particularly with endocardial cushion defect (ECD) and tricuspid atresia.
   b. Right bundle branch block (RBBB).

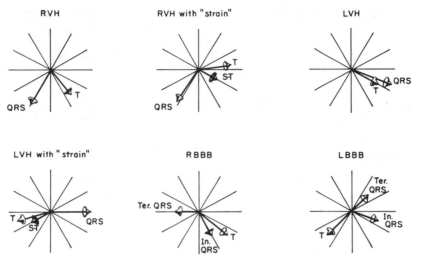

FIG 3–3.
Characteristic disorders of QRS and T axes associated with major categories of hypertrophy and conduction disturbances. Magnitudes of the vectors are not proportional. Terminal and initial QRS are abbreviated *"Ter."* and *"In."* (From Guntheroth WG: *Pediatric Electrocardiography.* Philadelphia, WB Saunders Co, 1965. Used by permission.)

QRS Duration

The QRS duration represents the time required for ventricular depolarization (see Fig 3–1). It is short in the young infant and increases with age (Table 3–2). The average QRS durations are:

Premature infants	0.04 second
Full-term infants	0.05 second
Children 1 to 3 years	0.06 second
Children more than 3 years	0.07 second
Adults	0.08 second

Since the QRS duration increases with a person's age, the definition of ventricular conduction disturbances (such as bundle branch block and Wolff-Parkinson-White syndrome) should vary with age. When the QRS duration is beyond the upper limit of normal for a given age, a ventricular conduction disturbance is present. In adults a QRS duration greater than 0.10 sec-

TABLE 3–2.
QRS Duration: Average (and Upper Limits) for Age

	0–1 mo	1–6 mo	6 mo–1 yr	1–3 yr	3–8 yr	8–12 yr	12–16 yr	Adult
Seconds	0.05(0.065)	0.05(0.07)	0.05(0.07)	0.06(0.07)	0.07(0.08)	0.07(0.09)	0.07(0.10)	0.08(0.10)

Modified from Guntheroth WG: *Pediatric Electrocardiography.* Philadelphia, WB Saunders Co, 1965. (Used by permission.)

ond is required for diagnosis of a bundle branch block, but in infants a duration of 0.08 second meets the requirements of a bundle branch block. There is no virtue in dividing bundle branch block into "complete" and "incomplete" in pediatric cases.

Abnormal QRS Duration

An *abnormally wide QRS duration* indicates an abnormal delay or an abnormal spread of the impulse through the ventricles and is a common finding in conditions grouped as ventricular conduction disturbances (see Chap. 5). Therefore, it is seen in the following conditions:

1. Bundle branch block, right or left.
2. Preexcitation (WPW syndrome).
3. Intraventricular block.
4. Arrhythmias of ventricular origin.
5. Implanted ventricular pacemaker.

QRS Amplitude

The most important diagnostic criteria of ventricular hypertrophy are abnormally large QRS voltages in the leads representing the respective ventricles. Normal and upper limits of normal R and S wave amplitudes of important leads are shown in Table 3–3.

Abnormal QRS Amplitude

1. *Abnormally large deflections,* either positive or negative, may indicate:
   a. Ventricular hypertrophy, right or left.
   b. Ventricular conduction disturbances such as:
      Right or left bundle branch block.
      Preexcitation.
      Intraventricular block.
      Artificial ventricular pacemaker.
2. *Low-voltage QRS complexes* (the limb lead deflections of less than 5 mm) are seen in:
   a. Myocarditis.
   b. Pericardial effusion (pericarditis).
   c. Chronic constrictive pericarditis.
   d. Hypothyroidism.
   e. Adults with thick chest wall.
   f. Normal newborn infants.

Q Wave

The Q wave is produced primarily by depolarization of the ventricular septum (see Fig 3–1). A Q wave is commonly present in leads I, II, III, and aVF and almost always present in V5 and V6. The Q wave is absent in V4R and V1 except for rare instances in the newborn infant.

The maximal Q amplitude in leads aVF, V5, and V6 is usually less than 5 mm in children of any age. The maximal Q wave amplitude in lead III may be as large as 5 to 8 mm in children (Table 3–4). The average Q wave duration is 0.02 second and normally does not exceed 0.03 second.

TABLE 3–3.

R Voltages According to Lead and Age: Mean (and Upper Limits)*

Lead	0–1 mo	1–6 mo	6 mo–1 yr	1–3 yr	3–8 yr	8–12 yr	12–16 yr	Young Adults
I	4 (8)	7 (13)	8 (16)	8 (16)	7 (15)	7 (15)	6 (13)	6 (13)
II	6 (14)	13 (24)	13 (27)	13 (23)	13 (22)	14 (24)	14 (24)	9 (25)
III	8 (16)	9 (20)	9 (20)	9 (20)	9 (20)	9 (24)	9 (24)	6 (22)
aVR	3 (7)	3 (6)	3 (6)	2 (6)	2 (5)	2 (4)	2 (4)	1 (4)
aVL	2 (7)	4 (8)	5 (10)	5 (10)	3 (10)	3 (10)	3 (12)	3 (9)
aVF	7 (14)	10 (20)	10 (16)	8 (20)	10 (19)	10 (20)	11 (21)	5 (23)
V4R	6 (12)	5 (10)	4 (8)	4 (8)	3 (8)	3 (7)	3 (7)	
V1	15 (25)	11 (20)	10 (20)	9 (18)	7 (18)	6 (16)	5 (16)	3 (14)
V2	21 (30)	21 (30)	19 (28)	16 (25)	13 (28)	10 (22)	9 (19)	6 (21)
V5	12 (30)	17 (30)	18 (30)	19 (36)	21 (36)	22 (36)	18 (33)	12 (33)
V6	6 (21)	10 (20)	13 (20)	12 (24)	14 (24)	14 (24)	14 (22)	10 (21)

S Voltages According to Lead and Age: Mean (and Upper Limits)*

Lead	0–1 mo	1–6 mo	6 mo–1 yr	1–3 yr	3–8 yr	8–12 yr	12–16 yr	Young Adults
I	5 (10)	4 (9)	4 (9)	3 (8)	2 (8)	2 (8)	2 (8)	1 (6)
V4R	4 (9)	4 (12)	5 (12)	5 (12)	5 (14)	6 (20)	6 (20)	
V1	10 (20)	7 (18)	8 (16)	13 (27)	14 (30)	16 (26)	15 (24)	10 (23)
V2	20 (35)	16 (30)	17 (30)	21 (34)	23 (38)	23 (48)	14 (36)	14 (36)
V5	9 (30)	9 (26)	8 (20)	6 (16)	5 (14)	5 (17)	5 (16)	
V6	4 (12)	2 (7)	2 (6)	2 (6)	1 (5)	1 (4)	1 (5)	1 (13)

*Voltages are measured in millimeters, when 1 mV = 10 mm paper.
Modified from Guntheroth WG: *Pediatric Electrocardiography*. Philadelphia, WB Saunders Co, 1965.

TABLE 3–4.

Q Voltages According to Lead and Age: Mean (and Upper Limits)*

Lead	0–1 mo	1–6 mo	6 mo–1 yr	1–3 yr	3–8 yr	8–12 yr	12–16 yr	Adult
III	2 (5)	3 (8)	3 (8)	3 (8)	1.5 (6)	1 (5)	1 (4)	0.5 (4)
aVF	2 (4)	2 (5)	2 (6)	1.5 (5)	1 (5)	1 (3)	1 (3)	0.5 (2)
V5	1.5 (5)	1.5 (4)	2 (5)	2 (6)	2 (6)	2 (4.5)	1 (4)	0.5 (3.5)
V6	1.5 (4)	1.5 (4)	2 (5)	2 (4.5)	1.5 (4.5)	1.5 (4)	1 (2.5)	0.5 (3)

*Voltages measured in millimeters, when 1 mV = 10 mm paper.
From Guntheroth WG: *Pediatric Electrocardiography*. Philadelphia, WB Saunders Co, 1965. (Used by permission.)

Abnormal Q Waves

1. *No Q waves in V6:*
   a. L-transposition of the great arteries ("congenitally corrected" TGA).
   b. Single ventricle.
   c. Mirror-image dextrocardia.
   d. Left bundle branch block.
2. *Q waves in V1:*
   a. Severe right ventricular hypertrophy.
   b. L-transposition of the great arteries.
   c. Single ventricle.
   d. Occasional normal newborns.

3. *Deep* (but not wide) *Q waves* are associated with:
   a. LVH of volume overload type (seen with VSD, single ventricle), but not common with LVH of pressure overload type.
   b. Occasionally RVH.
   c. Combined ventricular hypertrophy (VSD + pulmonary hypertension).
   d. Myocardial disease characterized by abnormal diastolic compliance (cardiomyopathy).
4. *Deep and wide Q waves* are seen in:
   a. Myocardial infarction.
   b. Myocardial fibrosis.
   c. Idiopathic hypertrophic subaortic stenosis (QS pattern in left precordial leads).

R/S Progression

In adults and children more than 3 years of age there is a smooth progression in the precordial leads from rS in V4R and V1, through RS in V2 and V3 and qRs in V4 through V6 *(adult R/S progression)*. In other words, there is a progressive increase in amplitude of the R wave toward V5 and a progressive decrease in amplitude of the S wave toward V6 (see Figs 2–5, 2–6, and 2–7). In infants in the first month of life, there may be *complete reversal* of the R/S progression, with a dominant R in V4R, V1, and V2 (the right precordial leads) and a dominant S in V5 and V6 (the left precordial leads). In children between 1 month and 2 to 3 years of age, *partial reversal* is usually present, with a dominant R in V1 as well as in V5 and V6.

Deviations from this age-dependent R/S progression may be associated with the following:

1. Ventricular hypertrophy.
2. Ventricular conduction disturbances.
3. Single ventricle.
4. Myocardial infarction.

R/S Ratio

An abnormal R/S ratio, either less than lower limit of normal (LLN) or greater than the upper limit of normal (ULN), is an important diagnostic criterion for ventricular hypertrophy (see Chap. 4, Hypertrophy). This ratio is a quantification of the concept of the R/S progression, but is manifested in specific leads.

In infants, because of the physiologic right ventricular dominance, the R/S ratio normally is large in the right precordial leads (RPLs: V1, V2), and the ratios are small in the left precordial leads (LPLs: V5, V6). In adults, because of the left ventricular dominance, the R/S ratios are small in the RLPs and the ratios are large in the LPLs (Table 3–5).

Abnormal R/S Ratios

R/S ratio >ULN in RPLs suggests RVH

<LLN in RPLs suggests LVH

R/S ratio >ULN in LPLs suugests LVH

<LLN in LPLs suggests RVH

Abnormal R/S ratios may also be seen in ventricular conduction disturbances (see Chap. 5) and myocardial infarction.

TABLE 3–5.

R/S Ratio According to Age: Mean, Lower, and Upper Limits of Normal

Lead	0–1 mo	1–6 mo	6 mo–1 yr	1–3 yr	3–8 yr	8–12 yr	12–16 yr	Adult
LLN*	0.5	0.3	0.3	0.5	0.1	0.15	0.1	0.0
V1 Mean	1.5	1.5	1.2	0.8	0.65	0.5	0.3	0.3
ULN†	19	S = 0	6	4	2	1	1	1
LLN	0.3	0.3	0.3	0.3	0.05	0.1	0.1	0.1
V2 Mean	1	1.2	1	0.8	0.5	0.5	0.5	0.2
ULN	3	4	4	1.5	1.5	1.2	1.2	2.5
LLN	0.1	1.5	2	3	2.5	4	2.5	2.5
V6 Mean	2	4	6	20	20	20	10	9
ULN	S = 0	S = 0	S = 0	S = 0	S = 0	S = 0	S = 0	S = 0

*Lower limits of normal.
†Upper limits of normal.
Modified from Guntheroth WG: *Pediatric Electrocardiography*. Philadelphia, WB Saunders Co, 1965. (Used by permission.)

ST SEGMENT

The ST segment occurs after ventricular depolarization (the QRS complex), and before ventricular repolarization (the T wave) (see Fig 3–1). The normal ST segment is horizontal and isoelectric (at the same level as the PQ and TP segments). In the limb leads, elevation or depression of the ST segment up to 1 mm is not necessarily abnormal. A shift of up to 2 mm is considered normal in the left precordial leads. No data are available on the normal ST segment duration, but an abnormally prolonged ST segment will result in prolongation of QT interval, for which normal values have been established.

Abnormal ST Segment (Elevated or Depressed)

1. Pericarditis.
2. Myocarditis.
3. Acute myocardial infarction or ischemia.
4. Hyperkalemia or hypokalemia.
5. Severe ventricular hypertrophy ("strain").
6. Ventricular aneurysm.
7. Drug effect (digitalis).
8. Intracranial pathology.

T WAVE

The T wave represents the ventricular repolarization process (see Fig 3–1). The amplitude of T wave is best measured in the left precordial leads. Although the T amplitude is influenced by many physiologic processes, the normal T amplitude is usually less than the following:

$$\begin{array}{lll}
\text{In V5:} & <1 \text{ year} & 11 \text{ mm} \\
 & >1 \text{ year} & 14 \text{ mm} \\
\text{In V6:} & <1 \text{ year} & 7 \text{ mm} \\
 & >1 \text{ year} & 9 \text{ mm}
\end{array}$$

After adolescence, the amplitude is generally less than before.

Abnormal T Waves

1. *Tall, peaked T waves* may be seen in:
   a. Hyperkalemia.
   b. LVH ("volume overload").
   c. Cerebrovascular accident, particularly hemorrhage.
   d. Posterior myocardial infarction (tall T in precordial leads).
2. *Flat or low T waves* may be seen in:
   a. Normal newborn infants.
   b. Hypothyroidism.
   c. Hypokalemia.
   d. Hyper- or hypoglycemia.
   e. Pericarditis.
   f. Myocarditis.
   g. Myocardial ischemia (hypoxemia, anemia, shock, etc.).
   h. Digitalis effect.

T Axis

The T axis represents the mean vector of ventricular repolarization (see Fig 3–1). The mean is +25 degrees with a range of −40 to +100 degrees in the first week of life. In a child 1 month of age, the T axis almost reaches the adult mean of +45 degrees (with a range of 0 to +90 degrees) (see Fig 3–2).

In the horizontal plane the T axis is also markedly anterior with a resulting upright T wave in V1 in the immediate postnatal period. Normally the T vector becomes posterior (negative T in V1) by the fourth day of life. Although there is a wide range of normal, the average T vector remains posterior (and leftward) for the first 4 or 5 years of life; it then becomes progressively more anterior (and leftward) in later years. In summary, the normal T vector in the horizontal plane is always oriented to the left at any age. It is usually posterior in children up to 5 years of age and is usually anterior in people more than 10 years of age. In children between 5 and 10 years of age it may be either anterior or posterior.

Abnormal T Axis

An abnormal T axis may be associated with the following (see also Fig 3–3):

1. Ventricular hypertrophy with "strain."
2. Bundle branch block.
3. Pericarditis.
4. Myocarditis.
5. Myocardial ischemia.
6. Ventricular arrhythmias.
7. Intracranial pathology.

QRS-T ANGLE

The QRS-T angle provides information on the normality of the ventricular repolarization process. It is a sensitive index of significant T wave abnormalities and is more reliable than the empirical observation of T wave changes in isolated leads.

In general, the QRS and T axes are similar, as indicated by their normal ranges shown in Figure 3–2. However, in early infancy the QRS-T angle normally may be wide. By the time a baby is 3 months of age, the mean QRS-T angle should be 30 degrees. In children more than 3 months of age, a QRS-T angle of more than 60 degrees may be abnormal, and one of more than 90 degrees is certainly abnormal.

A wide QRS-T angle is less significant if the T axis is in the normal quadrant (0 to +90 degrees) than if the T axis is outside this quadrant. Normally, the T axis should remain in the normal quadrant (0 to +90 degrees), regardless of the QRS axis.

Abnormal QRS-T Angle

An abnormally wide QRS-T angle is seen in the following (see also Fig 3–3):

1. Severe right or left ventricular hypertrophy ("strain").
2. Ventricular conduction disturbances.
3. Myocardial dysfunction (metabolic or ischemic).

QT INTERVAL

The QT interval represents the time required for both ventricular depolarization (QRS duration) and ventricular repolarization (to the end of the T wave) (see Fig 3–1). The QT interval varies with heart rate but not with age, except in infancy. Therefore, the QT interval must be interpreted in relation to the heart rate (corrected QT interval, QTc). One may use either a table of averages and upper limits of normal (Table 3–6) or Bazett's formula.

$$\text{Bazett's formula: QT}c = \frac{\text{QT measured}}{\sqrt{\text{RR } interval}}$$

According to Bazett's formula, the QTc should not exceed 0.44 second, except in infants. The QTc of up to 0.49 second may be normal for the first six months of life. The calculation should be based on a steady state.

U waves are small, positive waves that occur toward the end of the T wave and should not be included in the QT measurement. The U waves are usually prominent in hypokalemia and may produce the appearance of a prolonged QTc, whereas the true QTc (without the U wave) is not prolonged.

TABLE 3–6.

Cycle Length, Heart Rate, and QT Interval Average (and Upper Limits)

Cycle Length (sec)	Heart Rate (per min)	Average QT (Upper Limit) (sec)	Cycle Length (sec)	Heart Rate (per min)	Average QT (Upper Limit) (sec)
1.50	40	0.45 (0.49)	0.85	70	0.36 (0.38)
1.40	43	0.44 (0.48)	0.80	75	0.35 (0.38)
1.30	46	0.43 (0.47)	0.75	80	0.34 (0.37)
1.25	48	0.42 (0.46)	0.70	86	0.33 (0.36)
1.20	50	0.41 (0.45)	0.65	92	0.32 (0.35)
1.15	52	0.41 (0.45)	0.60	100	0.31 (0.34)
1.10	55	0.40 (0.44)	0.55	109	0.30 (0.33)
1.05	57	0.39 (0.43)	0.50	120	0.28 (0.31)
1.00	60	0.39 (0.42)	0.45	133	0.27 (0.29)
0.95	63	0.38 (0.41)	0.40	150	0.25 (0.28)
0.90	67	0.37 (0.40)	0.35	172	0.23 (0.26)

From Guntheroth WG: *Pediatric Electrocardiography*. Philadelphia, WB Saunders Co, 1965. (Used by permission.)

Abnormal QT Intervals

1. *Prolonged QT interval* may be seen in:
   a. Hypocalcemia.
   b. Myocarditis, rheumatic or viral.
   c. Long QT syndrome: Jervell and Lange-Nielsen syndrome and Romano-Ward syndrome.
   d. Head injury or cerebrovascular accidents.
   e. Diffuse myocardial disease.
   f. Quinidine, procainamide, etc.
2. *Short QT interval* may be seen in:
   a. Hypercalcemia (due to short ST segment).
   b. Digitalis effect.

REVIEW QUESTIONS

Answer the following questions either "true" or "false."

1. The QRS duration in a normal newborn infant is 0.10 second.	True	False
2. The PR interval increases with decreasing heart rate and increasing age.	True	False
3. A normal P axis ranges from 0 to +90 degrees in people of any age.	True	False
4. The mean QRS axis in a week-old newborn infant is between 0 and +90 degrees.	True	False
5. The QT interval increases with increasing age.	True	False
6. A heart rate of 130 per minute in a newborn infant is tachycardia.	True	False
7. An upright P wave in lead III is an indication of sinus rhythm.	True	False
8. The QRS duration of a normal newborn infant is less than that of an adult.	True	False
9. The amplitude of the T wave increases progressively with age, up to adolescence.	True	False

Answers may be found on page 238.

CHAPTER 4

Hypertrophy

Owing to the nature of heart disease in children, i.e., structural abnormalities with volume and/or pressure overload, hypertrophy is probably the most common abnormality seen in pediatric electrocardiograms (ECGs). In order to recognize hypertrophy, one must become familiar with the normal data, particularly normal QRS voltages and normal ranges of the QRS and T axes. Reference to these normal data, presented in Chapter 3, is frequently necessary for accurate interpretation of pediatric ECGs.

ATRIAL HYPERTROPHY

Since the P wave represents atrial electrical activity, abnormalities in P waves are expected to occur in atrial hypertrophy. However, unlike ventricular hypertrophy, in which QRS axis deviation usually occurs, there is no shift of the P axis in the frontal plane in atrial hypertrophy. The changes with atrial hypertrophy are increases in the amplitude and/or duration of the P wave.

Figure 4–1 will help in understanding the anticipated changes in atrial hypertrophy. The right atrium (RA) is depolarized earlier than the left atrium (LA) because of proximity of the sinoatrial (SA) node to the RA. The vector of RA depolarization is directed anteriorly (and inferiorly), whereas that of the LA is directed leftward (and inferiorly). When seen from the positive pole of lead II (on the hexaxial reference system, see Fig 1–14), the mean P axis is about +60 degrees and produces a positive P wave that is believed to consist of an early right atrial (upright) and a terminal left atrial (upright) component. When seen from the V1 electrode, the P wave consists of an early right atrial (upright) component and a terminal left atrial (downward) component. Changes resulting from hypertrophy of either or both of the atria can be deduced and are shown diagrammatically in Figure 4–1. This is a simplified concept and does not cover all clinical situations, of course.

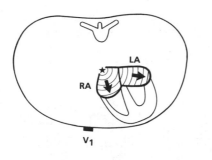

	NORMAL	RAH	LAH	CAH
II	RA LA	RA · LA	RA · LA	RA · LA
V₁	RA · LA	RA · LA	RA · LA	RA · LA

FIG 4–1.
Cross-sectional diagram of the atria shows the direction of atrial depolarization, and anticipated P wave changes are presented for right atrial hypertrophy *(RAH)*, left atrial hypertrophy *(LAH)*, and combined atrial hypertrophy *(CAH)*.

Criteria for Atrial Hypertrophy

Right Atrial Hypertrophy (RAH).—Called "p-pulmonale" since it is frequently associated with cor pulmonale, RAH produces tall P waves, 3 mm or greater, in any lead. This pattern is present most often in lead II and occasionally in V1 and V2 (Fig 4–2).

Left Atrial Hypertrophy (LAH).—Called "p-mitrale" because of its frequent association with mitral valve disease, LAH produces prolongation of the P duration, 0.10 second or greater, in any lead. In infants less than 12 months of age, a P duration of 0.08 second or greater may satisfy the criterion. A broad and notched P wave in the limb leads is characteristic of LAH. Often the P wave is diphasic in V1 with a negative, prolonged, terminal segment. Even in the presence of notched or diphasic P waves, as described above, prolongation of the P duration is a requirement for LAH (see Fig 4–2).

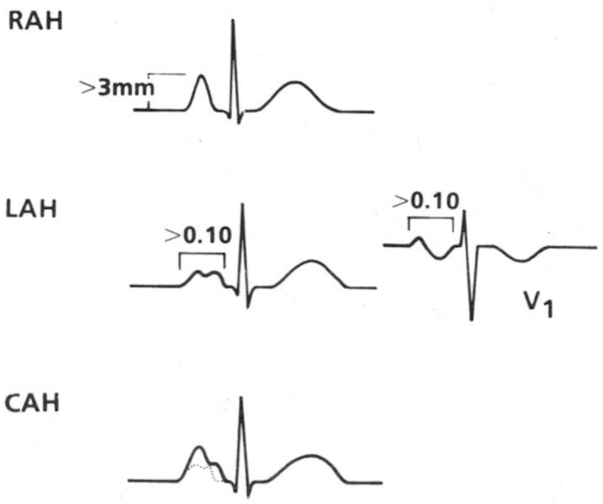

RAH

>3mm

FIG 4–2.
Criteria for atrial hypertrophy.

LAH

>0.10   >0.10

V₁

CAH

Combined Atrial Hypertrophy (CAH).—Combined atrial hypertrophy produces a combination of increases in amplitude and duration of the P waves (see Fig 4–2).

Example of RAH (Fig 4–3)

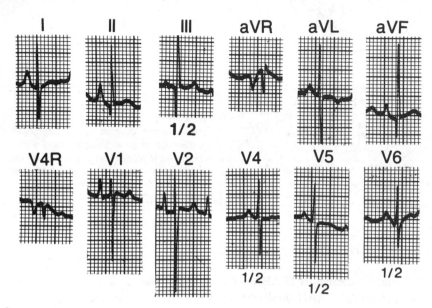

FIG 4–3.
Tracing from a 4-month-old boy with pulmonary atresia with hypoplastic RV and patent ductus arteriosus.

In Figure 4–3, the P waves are abnormally tall in many limb and precordial leads. The P wave is 3.5 mm in lead I, 5 mm in lead II, and 4 mm in V1. The P waves are also abnormally tall in V4 and V6, considering their ½ standardization. Negative P waves are 3 mm deep in leads aVR and V4R. Left ventricular hypertrophy (LVH) with possible additional right ventricular hypertrophy (RVH) is also present (see below ventricular hypertrophy).

Interpretation: RAH, LVH, and possible additional RVH.

Example of LAH (Fig 4—4)

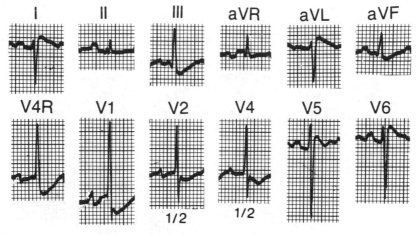

FIG 4—4.
Tracing from a 3-week-old girl with severe congenital mitral stenosis.

In Figure 4—4, the P wave amplitude is normal, but the P wave duration is prolonged, being most clearly visible in V1 (probably factitiously prolonged to 0.13 second). In this lead the P waves are diphasic with a long negative terminal portion. Diphasic P waves are also seen in V4R and V2, with P duration of 0.09 second, which is abnormally long in a 3-week-old infant, confirming LAH. The P waves are broad and notched in leads I, II, aVF, V5, and V6. A negative notched P wave is present in aVR. Other abnormalities in this tracing are deep S waves in leads I, V5, and V6, and tall R waves in V4R and V1, indicative of right ventricular hypertrophy (RVH).

Interpretation: LAH, and RVH.

Example of CAH (Fig 4–5)

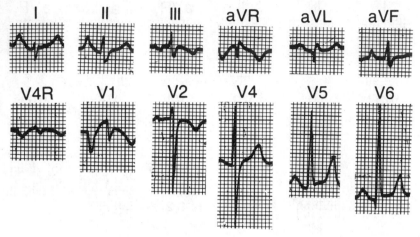

FIG 4–5.
Tracing from a 7-year-old boy with tricuspid atresia.

In Figure 4–5, the P waves are not only tall but are also wide. The P amplitude is 4.0 mm in leads I and II, indicating RAH. The P duration is abnormally long, approximately 0.12 second, best seen in lead I, in V4R, and in the left precordial leads. The shape of the P wave in lead I is characteristic of CAH (see Fig 4–2).

Interpretation: CAH, and LVH.

VENTRICULAR HYPERTROPHY

Ventricular hypertrophy produces abnormalities in one or more of the following areas, each of which will be discussed in detail: (1) the QRS axis; (2) the QRS voltages; (3) the R/S ratio; (4) ventricular repolarization ("strain" pattern) in severe hypertrophy; (5) the QRS duration; and (6) miscellaneous nonspecific changes.

Changes in the QRS Axis

In conjunction with the QRS voltage changes (discussed on next page), the QRS axis is usually directed toward the ventricle that is hypertrophied. There is right axis deviation (RAD) with right ventricular hypertrophy (RVH). Although the QRS axis tends to be more leftward than is normal for the patient's age with left ventricular hypertrophy (LVH), marked left axis deviation (LAD) is rare and is usually associated with conduction disturbance rather than with LVH (see Fig 3–2 for the normal ranges and Fig 3–3 for abnormal axis deviation). In concentric LVH (thickening without dilatation), the QRS axis frequently is almost vertical, near +90 degrees.

Changes in the QRS Voltages

With ventricular hypertrophy there is an increase in the voltage of the QRS complex in the leads that reflect the respective ventricle. Let us now consider the anatomical reasons for the changes that occur with RVH and LVH.

In the frontal plane (Fig 4–6,A), the LV mass lies to the left and inferior to the cardiac "center of gravity," and the RV lies to the right and inferior. Accordingly, the left and/or inferior vector represents LV force and the rightward vector represents RV force. Therefore, in left ventricular hypertrophy, the R wave voltage will be increased in leads I, II, aVL, aVF, and sometimes III. By the same token, in right ventricular hypertrophy, the R wave voltage will be increased in aVR and III, and the S voltage will be increased in leads I and aVL (see Fig 4–6,A).

In the horizontal projection (Fig 4–6,B), the RV occupies the right and anterior aspect and the LV the left and posterior aspect of the ventricular mass. Therefore, the RV force is represented by the R waves of V4R, V1, and V2, and the S waves of V5 and V6. The LV force is represented by the R waves of V5 and V6 and by the S waves of V4R, V1, and V2.

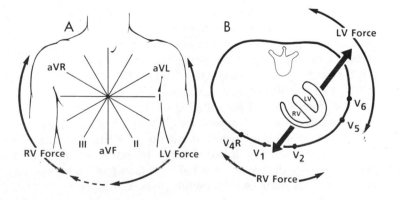

FIG 4–6.
Diagrammatic representation of left and right ventricular forces on the frontal projection or hexaxial reference system **(A)** and the horizontal plane **(B)**.

Tall R waves in V4R, V1, and V2 or deep S waves in V5 and V6 are seen in RVH, and tall R waves in V5 and V6 and/or deep S waves in V4R, V1, and V2 are seen in LVH.

In RVH, therefore, the abnormal deviation of RV force may be rightward and/or anterior. When this deviation is both anterior and rightward, the diagnosis of RVH is more secure than when there is deviation only in the anterior direction. In other words, only anterior deviation occurs with mild RVH, whereas the displacement is in both anterior and rightward directions with moderate RVH. Naturally, the R waves in V1 reflect rightward *and* anterior force, and the increased R voltage in V1 is a reliable sign of RVH.

An abnormally deep S wave in lead I is a reliable and reproducible sign of RVH. However, abnormally deep S waves in V5 and/or V6 in the absence of abnormal rightward forces in other leads are relatively weak criteria of RVH. This is sometimes caused by imprecise placement of chest lead electrodes, and may be seen in otherwise normal children.

Because of inconsistency of left axis deviation in LVH, abnormally large leftward and posterior or inferior forces are the important criteria of LVH. Pressure overload lesions, such as aortic stenosis, often manifest themselves by abnormally large inferior (tall R waves in II, III, and aVF) and posterior (deep S in V1 and V2) force with little leftward force, whereas volume overload lesions, such as patent ductus arteriosus or ventricular septal defect, manifest themselves by increased leftward force (tall R waves in V5 and V6).

It is important to point out, however, that abnormally tall R voltage in V6 alone (without abnormally tall R waves in V5) is a relatively weak criterion of LVH. This is seen often in otherwise normal children because of imprecise positioning of the V6 electrode too close to the position of the V5 electrode (see Fig 9–14, for example).

So far we have examined the leads that would show abnormally large voltages for each ventricle. The next question is: What voltage level is abnormally large? Most books on adult ECGs give a few simple numbers to remember. For example, if the sum of the amplitudes of S in V1 and R in V5 or V6 is greater than 45 mm, a diagnosis of LVH is suggested. This approach is logically unsound for interpreting pediatric ECGs, since infants and young children have continually changing QRS voltages as they grow. A logical approach is to compare the observed voltages with the available normal data for that particular age and see if the observed voltages are within normal limits or are beyond the upper limit of normal. The more leads with abnormally large QRS voltages, the more probable is ventricular hypertrophy.

Abnormal R/S Ratio

Let us now consider the concept of R/S ratio. The R/S ratio represents the relative force of opposing electromotive force in a given lead. In ventricular hypertrophy one may see an increase in the absolute voltage for the corresponding ventricle, but one may also see only a change in the R/S ratio if there is almost perfect cancellation of the opposing electromotive forces. An increase in the R/S ratio in the RPL (V4R, V1, and V2) suggests RVH, and a decrease in the R/S ratio in these leads suggests LVH. By the same token, an increase in the R/S ratio in the LPL (V5 and V6) suggests LVH, and a decrease in the ratio suggests RVH. The mean, upper, and lower limits of normal are given in Table 3–5.

An increase in the R/S ratio of V1 beyond the ULN represents a relative increase in both rightward and anterior force and is an important criterion of RVH, particularly if the R wave is over 5 mm in amplitude. When the R wave voltage is less than 5 mm, an abnormally increased R/S ratio has less significance. An R/S ratio less than 1 in V6 in children more than 1 month of age is very unusual and is another useful criterion of RVH.

"Strain" Pattern

"Strain" is a useful term signifying abnormal ventricular repolarization associated with severe ventricular hypertrophy. This is usually a result of relative ischemia of the hypertrophied myocardium. The "strain" pattern is present when there is a wide QRS-T angle with the T axis outside the normal range in the frontal plane (outside the 0 to +90 degree quadrant). As long as the T axis remains in the normal quandrant (0 to +90 degrees), a wide QRS-T angle alone may only indicate a possible "strain" pattern for either LVH or RVH (Figs 3–3 and 4–7).

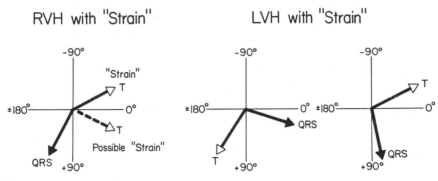

FIG 4–7.
Locations of QRS and T axes in ventricular hypertrophy with "strain."

In *RVH with "strain,"* the QRS axis is usually shifted more to the right than is normal for the patient's age, and the T axis (and the ST segment) is usually leftward and posterior, away from the direction of the QRS axis (see Figs 3–3 and 4–7). Therefore, in a clear-cut case of RVH with "strain," the QRS-T angle is wide (greater than 90 degrees), and the T axis is in the left upper quadrant (0 to −90 degrees), with inverted T waves in aVF. If the QRS-T angle is equal to or greater than 90 degrees, but the T axis is still in the normal quadrant, in the presence of RVH, a diagnosis of RVH with *possible* "strain" is appropriate (see Fig 4–7). As long as the frontal plane (limb leads) shows the QRS-T angle to be less than 90 degrees and the T axis to be in the normal quadrant, the mere presence of a wide QRS-T angle in the horizontal plane (the T wave opposite to the main QRS deflection in V1 and V2) is not evidence of "strain," since the T vector may normally be either anterior or posterior during childhood.

The principles discussed above for the "strain" pattern with RVH also apply for *LVH with "strain."* The presence of a wide QRS-T angle with the T vector in an abnormal quadrant in the presence of LVH indicates LVH with "strain." Characteristically, the T axis is in the right lower quadrant with inverted T waves in lead I, and the QRS axis is somewhat more leftward than normal for the patient's age, although still in the normal (0 to +90 degrees) quadrant (see Figs 3–3 and 4–7). When the LVH is manifested by a strong inferior force (rather than leftward force), the T axis may be in the left upper quadrant (0 to −90 degrees) with inverted T waves in aVF in the presence of a wide QRS-T angle. Shift of the ST segment may occur in the same direction as the T vector change (see Fig 4–7).

Prolongation of QRS Duration

The QRS duration may be mildly prolonged in ventricular hypertrophy, primarily as the result of increased muscle mass, which will predictably increase the total time for depolarization of all the muscle mass. Since prolongation of the QRS duration is also found with ventricular conduction disturbance (such as bundle branch block, Wolff-Parkinson-White syndrome, or intraventricular block), this creates some difficulties in a situation in which abnormally tall (or deep) QRS forces are seen in association with wide QRS duration (see Chap. 5 for further discussion).

Ventricular activation time (VAT) (or the time of onset of the "intrinsicoid deflection") is the duration between the onset of the QRS and the peak of the R wave (QR interval). Prolongation of the VAT, when the total duration of the QRS complex is normal, has been shown to be present in adults with ventricular hypertrophy. The concept of the VAT has limited values both on theoretical and practical grounds. Delineation of the VAT is more difficult in infants and children who normally have shorter QRS duration than do adults. Therefore, an increased VAT is not a reliable criterion of ventricular hypertrophy in infants and children.

Miscellaneous Nonspecific Changes

RVH

1. A q wave in V1 (either in the form of qR or qRs) is a suggestive sign of RVH. It is, however, nonspecific, because a qR pattern may occur in about 10% of normal neonates. One should make sure it is not an rsR′ with a very small or isoelectric r wave, giving an erroneous suggestion of qR pattern in V1. A q wave in V1 also occurs in L-TGA and single ventricle.

2. An upright T in V1 in patients more than 3 days of age: The T wave in V1 almost always becomes negative by 3 days of age. If not, RVH is probable. This is, however, nonspecific, since the upright T wave in V1 can be due to LVH with inverted T wave in V6 ("strain"), and some normal infants may have upright T in V1 as well.

LVH

1. Deep Q waves in V5 and V6 (5 mm or more) have been said to suggest left ventricular diastolic (or volume) overload. Many patients with large ventricular septal defect (VSD) have deep Q waves in V5 and V6 but they are not specific for that lesion. Since the Q wave represents early ventricular depolarization, deep Q waves in the LPL may indicate septal hypertrophy.

2. Tall T waves in V5 and V6 have been considered as evidence of LV diastolic or volume overload. However, these are also seen in otherwise normal children and are therefore nonspecific.

Combined Ventricular Hypertrophy

Many forms of congenital heart disease produce volume and/or pressure overload on both ventricles with resulting hypertrophy of both ventricles. Electrocardiographic evidence of combined ventricular hypertrophy (CVH) may be manifested in several ways, and sometimes is difficult to diagnose because of overlap with the normal ECG, particularly in children 6 months to 3 years of age.

When there are abnormally large voltages for both ventricles, satisfying criteria for both RVH and LVH, the diagnosis of CVH is clear-cut. However, because of cancellation of opposing forces, the voltage criteria for the hypertrophy of both ventricles may not be present. A common situation is that in which positive voltage criteria for hypertrophy of one ventricle are coupled with a relatively large (yet within the normal limit) force for the other ventricle. This is due to a *partial* cancellation of opposing forces. If there is, however, an almost *perfect* cancellation of opposing forces, one may see an ECG in which all the voltages are within normal limits in a child with an unequivocal biventricular hypertrophy. Another situation is the Katz-Wachtel phenomenon, in which large diphasic QRS complexes are present in two or more limb leads and in the mid-precordial leads (V2 through V5). This phenomenon suggests CVH if the voltages are greater than or close to the upper limit of normal (ULN) (see Table 3–3). Large equiphasic QRS complexes in the precordial leads alone are weak criteria, since many normal infants have such QRS complexes (see Chap. 2, Figs 2–3 and 2–4). It is easy to understand why the QRS vector directed strongly both leftward *and* rightward as well as anteriorly *and* posteriorly suggests CVH.

Criteria for Right Ventricular Hypertrophy (Summary)

1. Right axis deviation for the patient's age (see Figs 3–2 and 3–3).
2. Increased rightward and anterior QRS vector. Abnormal QRS forces rightward *and* anteriorly are stronger evidence of RVH than abnormal forces rightward or anteriorly alone.
   a. R in V4R, V1, V2, or aVR greater than the ULN for the patient's age.
   b. S in I or V6 greater than the ULN for the patients's age.
3. Abnormal R/S ratio in favor of the right ventricle (in the absence of bundle branch block).
   a. R/S ratio in V1 and V2 greater than the ULN for age.
   b. R/S ratio in V6 less than 1 after one month of age.
4. Upright T in V1 in patients more than 3 days of age, provided that the T is upright in the LPLs (V5, V6). Upright T in V1 is not necessarily abnormal in patients more than 6 years of age.
5. A q wave in V1 (qR or qRs patterns) is suggestive of RVH. (Make sure that there is not a small r in an rsR′ configuration.)
6. In the presence of RVH, a wide QRS-T angle with the T axis outside the normal range, usually in the 0 to −90 degree-quadrant, indicates "strain" pattern (see Figs 3–3 and 4–7).

In general, the greater the number of positive, independent criteria, the greater the probability of an abnormal degree of RVH.

RVH in the Newborn

The diagnosis of RVH in newborn infants is particularly difficult because of the normal dominance of the RV during that period of life. The following clues, however, are helpful in the diagnosis of RVH in newborn infants.

1. Pure R wave (with no S) in V1 greater than 10 mm.
2. R in V1 greater than 25 mm, or R in aVR greater than 8 mm.
3. A qR pattern in V1 (also seen in 10% of healthy newborn infants).
4. Upright T in V1 in neonates more than 3 days of age (with upright T wave in V6) is suggestive of RVH. (Upright T in V1 with negative T in V6 may often be seen in conditions that produce T vector changes (see Chap. 3) without RVH, such as myocarditis and myocardial ischemia).
5. Right axis deviation greater than +180 degrees.

Example 1 (Fig 4–8)

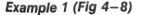

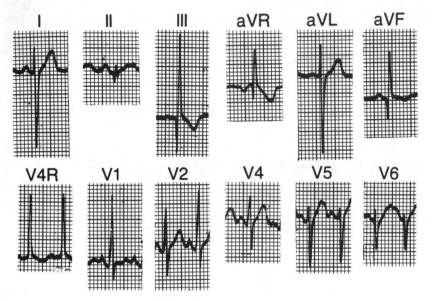

FIG 4–8.
Tracing from a 10-month-old child with severe tetralogy of Fallot.

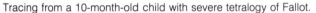

In Figure 4–8, the QRS axis is +150 degrees. There is RAD for the patient's age. The T axis is −10 degrees. The QRS-T angle is abnormally wide (160 degrees) with the T axis in an abnormal quadrant. The QRS duration is 0.06 second (normal). The PR interval is 0.12 second. The R waves in III (22 mm) and aVR (9 mm) and the S waves in I (19 mm) and V6 (8 mm) are abnormally large, indicating RVH. The R/S ratios in V1 and V2 are abnormally large, and the ratio in V6 is smaller than the LLN (see Table 3–5), all of which indicate RVH.

Interpretation: RVH with "strain."

Example 2 (Fig 4–9)

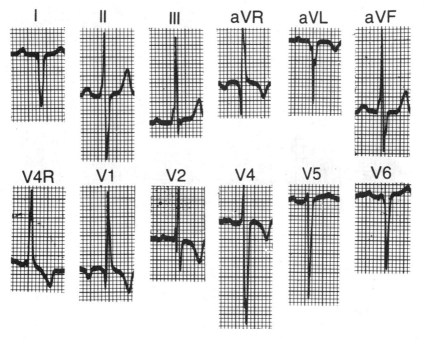

FIG 4–9.
Tracing from a 9-year-old boy with D-transposition of the great arteries, after a Blalock-Taussig shunt for pulmonary stenosis.

In Figure 4–9, the QRS axis is +150 degrees, beyond the ULN for the patient's age. The QRS duration is 0.07 second (normal) and the PR interval is 0.18 second. The S waves in leads I, V5, and V6, and the R wave in aVR are all beyond the ULN, indicating RVH. A q wave in V1 is also suggestive of RVH. The R/S ratios in V1 and V2 are abnormally large, and the ratio in V6 is abnormally small, again indicating RVH. The T axis is +80 degrees (in the normal quadrant) with a QRS-T angle of 70 degrees. Although the T waves in precordial leads are directed opposite to the mean QRS vector, indicating a wide QRS-T angle in the horizontal plane, the T vector may normally be anterior or posterior in a person of this age (see Chap. 3). Therefore, the "strain" pattern is not present.

Interpretation: RVH.

Example 3 (Fig 4−10)

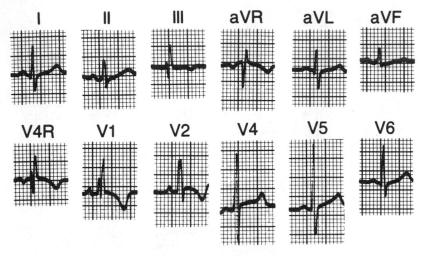

FIG 4−10.
Tracing from a 9-year-old boy with moderate pulmonary valve stenosis.

In Figure 4−10, the QRS axis is +50 degrees, which is normal. All the voltages are within normal limits. The only abnormalities are the R/S ratios in V1 (9) and V2 (4), which are abnormally large (ULN: 1.0 and 1.2, respectively). Although there is an rsR′ pattern in V4R and V1, the QRS duration is not prolonged (0.07 second in this case) and there is no terminal slurring of the QRS complex. Therefore, this is a case of mild RVH rather than right bundle branch block (see Chap. 5 for bundle branch blocks).

Interpretation: Mild RVH.

Criteria for Left Ventricular Hypertrophy (Summary)

1. Left axis deviation for the patient's age (see Figs 3−2 and 3−3).
2. QRS voltages in favor of the left ventricle (LV) (abnormal QRS voltages inferiorly, leftward and/or posteriorly):
   a. R in I, II, III, aVL, aVF, V5, or V6 greater than the ULN.
   b. S in V1 or V2 greater than the ULN.
   Pressure overload (e.g., aortic stenosis) is often reflected in tall R waves in II, III, and aVF, whereas volume overload (e.g., patent ductus arteriosus [PDA]) is reflected in V5 and V6.
3. Abnormal R/S ratio in favor of the LV:
   a. R/S ratio in V1 and V2 less than the lower limit of normal (LLN) for the patient's age.
4. Q in V5 and V6, 5 mm or more, coupled with tall symmetrical T waves in the same leads (suggestive of LVH), so-called LV diastolic overload.
5. In the presence of LVH, a wide QRS-T angle with the T axis outside the normal range indicates "strain" pattern. This is manifested by flat or inverted T waves in lead I or aVF (see Fig 4−7).

The greater the number of positive, independent criteria, the greater the probability of an abnormal degree of LVH.

Example 1 (Fig 4-11)

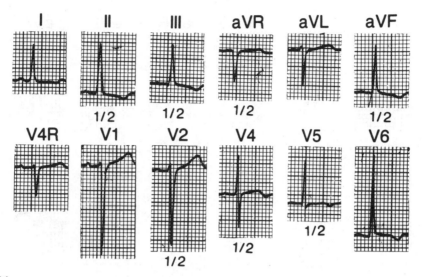

FIG 4-11.
Tracing from a 14-year-old girl with congenital aortic stenosis.

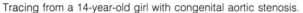

In Figure 4-11, the QRS axis is approximately +70 degrees (note ½ standardization markers in aVF and others). The T axis is -70 degrees (in an abnormal quadrant) with a wide QRS-T angle of 140 degrees. The R waves in leads II (25 mm), aVF (25 mm), and V5 (42 mm) are clearly beyond the ULN. The R in V6 and S in V2 are large but still within the normal limits. Therefore, we have voltage criteria for LVH and a wide QRS-T angle with the T axis in an abnormal quadrant, justifying the diagnosis of LVH with "strain."

Interpretation: LVH with "strain."

Example 2 (Fig 4—12)

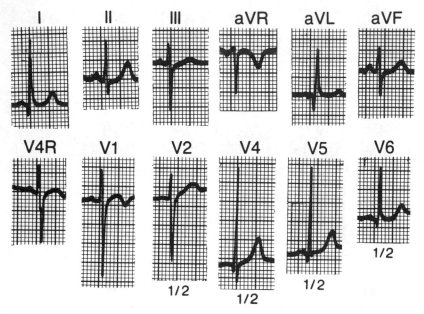

FIG 4—12.
Tracing from a 4-year-old boy with moderate ventricular septal defect.

In Figure 4—12, the QRS axis is 0 degrees, more leftward than normal for the patient's age. The T axis is +50 degrees with the QRS-T angle of 50 degrees. The R waves in I (17 mm), aVL (12 mm), V5 (44 mm), and V6 (27 mm) are beyond the upper limits of normal, indicating abnormal LV force. The S waves in V1 and V2 are within normal limits. The R/S ratios are also normal.

Interpretation: LVH.

Criteria for Combined Ventricular Hypertrophy (Summary)

1. Positive voltage criteria for right *and* left ventricular hypertrophy (in the absence of bundle branch block or preexcitation).
2. Positive voltage criteria for RVH *or* LVH and relatively large voltages for the other ventricle.
3. Large equiphasic QRS complexes in two or more of the limb leads and in the mid-precordial leads (V2 through V5), called the Katz-Wachtel phenomenon.

Example 1 (Fig 4–13)

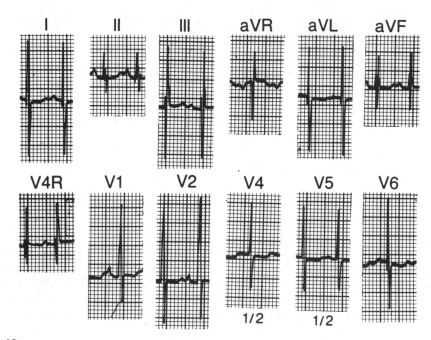

FIG 4–13.
Tracing from a 2-month-old infant with large-shunt VSD, PDA, and severe pulmonary hypertension.

In Figure 4–13, there are two distinct QRS vectors: initially leftward and terminally rightward. The QRSi is −10 degrees (see Fig 1–10,B); the net amplitude of the initial QRS of I = (−1) + (+15) = +14, and that of aVF = (+3) + (−5) = −2. The QRSt is +150 (I = −14; aVF = +9). The S waves in I and V6 are abnormally deep and the R in V1 is slightly beyond the ULN, suggesting RVH. In addition, the leftward voltages are also abnormal with the R waves in leads I and aVL beyond the ULN. The presence of large diphasic complexes in limb leads (I, III, aVR, aVL) and in the left precordial leads are characteristic of CVH (Katz-Wachtel phenomenon).

Interpretation: CVH.

Example 2 (Fig 4–14)

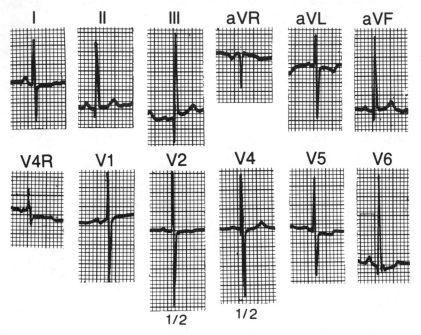

FIG 4–14.
Tracing from a 3-month-old infant with large ventricular septal defect and patent ductus arteriosus who received digoxin for congestive heart failure.

In Figure 4–14, the QRS axis is +80 degrees. The T vector is +90 degrees. The R in V6 and the S in V2 are beyond the ULN, suggesting LVH. The R in V2 is at the ULN. In other words, there is an abnormally large force directed not only to the left (R in V6) and posteriorly (S in V2), suggesting LVH, but also anteriorly (R in V2), suggesting additional RVH. The Katz-Wachtel phenomenon is present in the mid-precordial leads (V1 through V5).

Interpretation: CVH (with left ventricular dominance).

Example 3 (Fig 4–15)

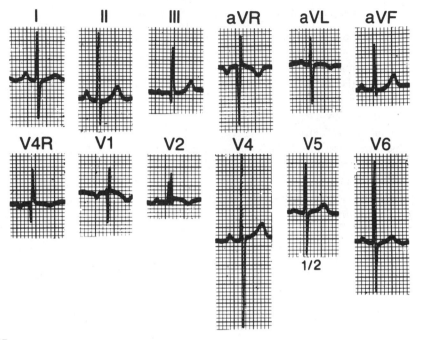

FIG 4–15.
Tracing from a 5-year-old girl with large ventricular septal defect and pulmonary artery banding.

In Figure 4–15, the QRS axis is +80 degrees. The S waves in I and V6 are abnormally deep and the R/S ratio in V2 is beyond the ULN, suggesting RVH. In addition, the leftward voltages are generous, with the R waves approaching the ULN in I and V6 (see criteria 2 for CHV). The presence of large diphasic QRS complexes in the limb leads (I, aVR, and aVL) (= Katz-Wachtel phenomenon) strongly suggests CVH.

Interpretation: CVH (with right dominance).

REVIEW QUESTIONS

In the following three questions, select as many answers as apply.

1. Which of the following are seen in RVH?
   a. R in V1 greater than ULN
   b. S in I greater than ULN
   c. Right axis deviation
   d. R/S ratio in V2 greater than the ULN
   e. R in aVL greater than ULN
   f. None of the above

2. Which are true with LVH?
   a. R in II or aVF greater than the ULN
   b. S in V2 greater than the ULN
   c. R/S ratio in V2 greater than the ULN
   d. Deep S in I
   e. Inverted T wave in V1
   f. None of the above

3. Which of the following deflections represent right ventricular force?
   a. S in lead I
   b. R in aVR
   c. R in aVL
   d. R in V5
   e. S in V2
   f. None of the above

Answer the following questions either "true" or "false."

4. The presence of P waves taller than 3 mm is an indication of left atrial hypertrophy.   True   False

5. The right ventricle occupies the right and anterior aspect of the ventricular mass.   True   False

6. An R/S ratio in V1 greater than the ULN indicates left ventricular dominance.   True   False

7. A q wave in V1 is suggestive of right ventricular hypertrophy.   True   False

8. The presence of the Katz-Wachtel phenomenon is suggestive of isolated right ventricular hypertrophy.   True   False

9. In a clear-cut case of RVH with "strain," the QRS-T angle is more than 90 degrees and the T axis is in the range of 0 to −90 degrees.   True   False

10. Diphasic P waves in V1 are an indication of left atrial hypertrophy, regardless of the duration of the P wave.   True   False

Answers may be found on page 238.

CHAPTER 5

Ventricular Conduction Disturbances

Ventricular conduction disturbances and chamber hypertrophies are the two most common forms of electrocardiographic abnormalities in pediatric patients. Right bundle branch block (RBBB) is the most common form of ventricular conduction disturbance, and the Wolff-Parkinson-White (WPW) syndrome has a unique clinical significance. These two forms will therefore be discussed in more detail than other types of conduction disturbances.

All conditions grouped under ventricular conduction disturbance have abnormal prolongation of QRS duration (Fig 5–1), with the exception of fascicular blocks. These conditions include RBBB, left bundle branch block (LBBB), WPW syndrome, intraventricular block, and implanted artificial ventricular pacemaker. In bundle branch block (right and left) and the artificial ventricular pacemaker the prolongation involves the terminal portion of the QRS complex (Fig 5–1,B). In the WPW syndrome the prolongation is in the initial portion of the QRS complex (Fig 5–1,C). In intraventricular block the prolongation is throughout the QRS complex (Fig 5–1,D). Occasional patients with ventricular hypertrophy will also have mild prolongation of the QRS complex.

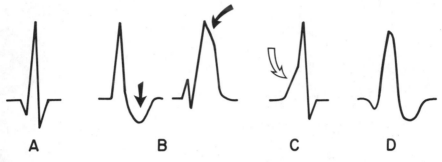

FIG 5–1.
Schematic diagram of three types of ventricular conduction disturbances. **A,** normal QRS complex. **B,** QRS complex in RBBB or premature ventricular contraction with prolongation of the terminal portion of the QRS complex (terminal slurring; *black arrows*). **C,** preexcitation with an initial slurring *(open arrow)* (delta wave). **D,** intraventricular block in which the prolongation of the QRS complex is throughout the QRS complex.

NORMAL VENTRICULAR DEPOLARIZATION

Let us briefly review the normal ventricular depolarization process in order to understand abnormal ventricular conduction. In a normal heart, shown in Figure 5–2, the septal depolarization is labeled "1," following which the right ventricle (RV) and left ventricle (LV) are depolarized almost simultaneously through the Purkinje system, labeled "2." Much of the opposing electromotive forces of the RV and LV cancel out each other, and the thicker ventricle (the LV in this case) will determine the final direction of the major vector. The ventricular depolarization process takes under 0.10 second in the adult and even less in children. Note that the direction of the septal depolarization is from left to right, producing Q waves in V6 (or the left precordial leads [LPLs]) and R waves in V1 (or the right precordial leads [RPLs]). This has an important application in understanding chamber localization, to be discussed in Chapter 8.

FIG 5–2.
Sequence of normal ventricular depolarization. Because of the direction of septal depolarization *(1),* there will be an initial R wave in *V1* and a q wave in *V6.* Simultaneous depolarization of both ventricles in opposite direction *(2)* results in QRS complexes of relatively small amplitude and of normal duration, with a dominant LV causing the rS in V1 and qR in V6.

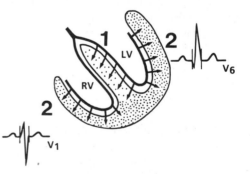

RIGHT BUNDLE BRANCH BLOCK (RBBB)

In true right bundle branch block (RBBB) the depolarization of the ventricular septum, labeled "1," and the LV, labeled "2" in Figure 5–3, is normal, but the RV is not depolarized directly through the Purkinje system. The RV is depolarized through the ventricular myocardium at a much slower rate (see "3" in the figure) since the conduction velocity through the ventricular myocardium is much slower than that through the Purkinje system (see Table 7–1). This slower rate of advance of depolarization results in prolongation of the terminal portion of the QRS complex, called *terminal "slurring"* (see Fig 5–3). The RV, which is depolarized last (shown in the figure as the darkest area), is located in the right and anterior aspect of the ventricular mass, and therefore the terminal slow depolarization (terminal slurring) is directed to the right and anteriorly. This is manifested by wide R' waves in the RPLs and aVR and slurred S waves in the LPLs and lead I (see Fig 5–3). The initial phase of ventricular depolarization remains normal. Therefore, in RBBB, the initial QRS vector (QRSi) remains in the normal quadrant; it is only the terminal QRS vector (QRSt) that changes in RBBB.

Since the LV is depolarized normally while unopposed by the RV depolarization, LV force greater than normal may result. At the time the RV is being depolarized ("3" in the figure) most of the LV has been depolarized and the RV potential is unopposed by the LV potential, resulting in a greater RV potential. Consequently, abnormally large forces for right and/or left ventricles may result even in the absence of actual hypertrophy of the ventricles.

Memorization of the QRS patterns, namely, wide and slurred S in I, V5, and V6, and slurred R' in aVR, V1, and V2, etc., is not necessary. All you need to remember is that the RBBB is manifested by terminal slurring directed to the *right* and *anteriorly,* reflecting the fact that the RV occupies the right and anterior aspect of the ventricular mass.

Right bundle branch block is the most common form of conduction disturbance in pediatric patients. However, in the common pediatric examples of RBBB the right bundle is actually intact. In lesions with right ventricular volume overload, the prolongation of ventricular activation and QRS duration is due to a longer pathway, conducting normally. Specifically, in atrial septal defect (ASD) the right ventricular volume may be three or four times the normal volume, and although conduction velocity is normal, the longer pathway requires a longer depolarization duration than that of the left ventricle. In a situation like this, the degree of QRS prolongation is usually mild. The terminology used to describe this type of QRS prolongation

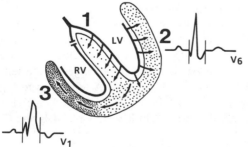

FIG 5–3.
Sequence of ventricular depolarization in RBBB. The septal depolarization *(1)* is normal with resulting Q in V6 and R in V1. The terminal slurring that is directed anteriorly and rightward produces rsR' pattern in V1 and qRS in V6. The amplitude of QRS may be abnormally large.

(without true "block") has been somewhat confusing, and all of the following terms have been used: incomplete RBBB, right ventricular conduction delay, mild RVH, and RV volume overload. In most cases RBBB occurs after open heart surgery that involves right ventriculotomy such as repair of ventricular septal defect or tetralogy of Fallot. The right ventriculotomy causes RBBB by disrupting the right ventricular subendocardial Purkinje network without injuring the main right bundle branch. These types of QRS prolongation without true "block" in the right bundle may not produce T wave changes. Of course, it is possible to surgically interrupt the right bundle branch during closure of the septal defect, but this is less common than the peripheral interruption with ventriculotomy. In addition to atrial septal defect and right ventriculotomy, RBBB is frequently seen in patients with Ebstein's anomaly and coarctation of the aorta in infants.

In adults, when the QRS duration is longer than 0.12 second it is called *complete RBBB*, and when the QRS duration is between 0.10 and 0.12 second it is called *incomplete RBBB*. However, division into complete and incomplete is generally arbitrary and is meaningless in children.

Formerly, some pediatricians regarded the RSR' pattern in V1 as evidence of RBBB. Although it is unusual to see this in adults, the RSR' pattern in V1 is a *normal* phenomenon in children provided that:

1. the QRS duration is not prolonged, and
2. the voltage of the primary or secondary R waves is not abnormally large.

If the QRS duration is prolonged, a conduction disturbance may be responsible for the RSR' pattern. The classic example is RBBB. If the R' wave is taller than the ULN for the patient's age and if QRS duration is normal, RVH is present. If the R' wave is abnormally tall with prolonged QRS duration, this is more likely RBBB rather than RVH (see criteria for RBBB further on). Evaluation of the occasional patient who shows mild but definite terminal slurring with the QRS duration still within normal limits for his age may be difficult. Such a patient probably should be considered normal rather than having RV conduction delay or incomplete RBBB. However, if the QRS duration is at the upper limits of normal (ULN), and there are other clinical grounds for suspecting an atrial septal defect, the ECG could properly be reported as "possible RBBB." It should be noted that RBBB may occur with no heart disease.

Let us examine why rsR' pattern and notched R or S waves in V1 are normal phenomena in infants and small children, employing vectorcardiographic QRS loops. As discussed in Chapter 1, complex changes take place in the horizontal QRS loop of the VCG from newborn period to adulthood. Fig 5–4,A is a normal QRS vector in the horizontal plane of a newborn with a clockwise loop, and Fig 5–4,F is a normal adult QRS vector with a counterclockwise loop. The right-anterior, clockwise QRS loop of the newborn gradually changes to the left-posterior, counterclockwise QRS loop of the adult. In order for Fig 5–4,A to change to Fig 5–4,F, the horizontal QRS loop has to go through various forms of complex loops (Fig 5–4,B through E), including those with one or more figure-of-eight loops (Fig 5–4,B and C) in early infancy.

In Fig 5–4,B, the initial loop is still clockwise but the terminal loop has assumed a counterclockwise direction, forming a figure-of-eight loop. The initial small clockwise half-loop (marked as *a*) produces an r wave. The loop then moves away from the V1 electrode to produce the downslope of the r wave, and continues to go beyond the isoelectric line (the dotted line drawn perpendicular to V1), producing a small s wave (marked as *b*). It then moves back toward the positive pole of V1, making a counterclockwise loop (marked as *c*). This produces a larger R′ wave before it moves back to the point of origin (E point). The end result is an rsR′ pattern in V1.

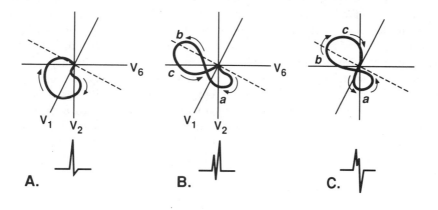

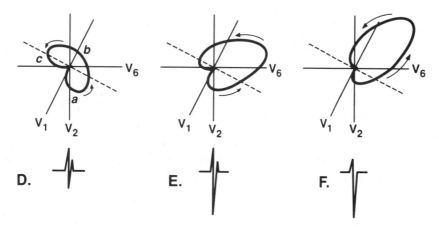

FIG 5–4.
Correlation between QRS patterns in V1 and vectorcardiographic loop in the horizontal plane as a function of age. In the newborn, the QRS loop is in the right-anterior quadrant, with the direction of inscription of the loop clockwise **(A).** In the adult, the QRS loop is in the left-posterior quadrant, counterclockwise in direction **(F).** In order for the newborn QRS loop **(A)** to change to the loop of the adult **(F),** the horizontal loop has to go through various stages, including those with one or more figure-of-eight loops **(B, C)** in early infancy. These loops **(B, C)** produce such QRS patterns as rsR′, RsrS′, or QRS complexes with notched R or S waves in V1. In the QRS loops seen in later infancy and childhood **(D, E),** the terminal portion of the loop crosses the broken line (isoelectric line for V1) and moves toward the positive pole of V1, producing an R′ wave. In the adult **(F),** the terminal portion of the QRS loop does not cross the isoelectric line, therefore no R′ wave is produced in V1.

In Fig 5–4,C, the initial half of the QRS loop is counterclockwise in direction and the latter half is clockwise. The initial loop (marked as *a*) produces an R wave. The latter half of the inital loop produces the downslope of the R wave but it does not reach the isoelectric line (the dotted line). It then moves back slightly toward the positive pole of V1 (marked as *b*), producing a notched R wave before it moves away to produce the downslope of the R wave and a larger S wave (marked as *c*). The end result is a notched R wave and an S wave in V1. If the initial counterclockwise loop *(a)* had reached the isoelectric line, Rr'S pattern would have resulted.

In Fig 5–4,D, the QRS loop is completely counterclockwise in direction as in the adult, but not as strongly to the left and posteriorly as in the adult. The loop then gradually increases its force to the left and posteriorly to assume the typical adult loop (Fig 5–4,F). In Figs 5–4,D and E, an RSr' pattern is recorded, because the terminal portion of the loop crosses the isoelectric line and moves toward the positive pole of V1. With vectorcardiographic correlation, it is easy to understand why the QRS complex in V1 may *normally* have notches in the R or S waves or an r' pattern. The QRS duration remains within normal limits even though the loop is complex; if the QRS duration is prolonged with an r' pattern, RBBB is present.

It is very unusual to see an rSr' pattern in V1 in adults. Fig 5–4,F is a typical horizontal QRS loop seen in the adult. The major force is to the left and posterior with a counterclockwise loop. Note that the terminal portion of the loop does not cross the isoelectric line; therefore, no r' is produced.

Criteria for RBBB (Summary)

1. Right axis deviation, at least for terminal portion of QRS (QRSt). Initial part of QRS (QRSi) is unchanged (see Fig 3–3).
2. QRS duration longer than the ULN for the patient's age (see Table 3–2).
3. Terminal slurring of the QRS complex directed to the right and usually, but not always, anteriorly (see Fig 3–3).
   a. Wide and slurred S in I, V5, and V6.
   b. Terminal, slurred R' in aVR and the RPLs (V4R, V1, and V2).
4. ST depression and T wave inversion are common in adults with RBBB, but not in children (see preceding text).
5. Asynchrony of the normally opposing electromotive force of each ventricle may result in a greater manifest potential for both ventricles. Therefore, the diagnosis of ventricular hypertrophy is insecure when either right or left BBB is present.

Example 1 (Fig 5–5)

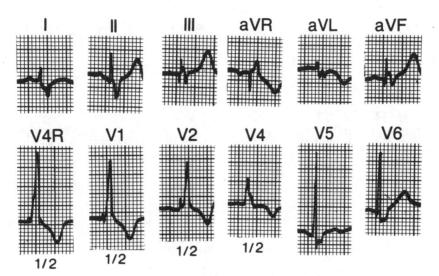

FIG 5–5.
Tracing from a 6-year-old boy who had corrective surgery for tetralogy of Fallot that involved right ventriculotomy for repair of ventricular septal defect and resection of infundibular narrowing.

In Figure 5–5, the QRS duration is increased (0.13 second); the maximal QRS duration at this age is 0.08 second (see Table 3–2). There is slurring of the terminal portion of the QRS complex, and this slurring is directed to the right (slurred S in I, V5, and V6, and slurred R in aVR) and anteriorly (slurred R in V4R, V1, and V2). The QRSt (terminal QRS axis) is approximately −160 degrees. The QRSi (initial QRS axis) is normal (+60 degrees). The T vector remains normal (+10 degrees). These findings satisfy the criteria for RBBB. The R waves in V4R, V1, and V2 are abnormally large, suggesting RVH. The R/S ratio in V1 is also abnormally increased. However, one cannot be sure of RVH since RBBB is present, even though the voltages are huge.

Interpretation: RBBB. Possible RVH.

Example 2 (Fig 5—6)

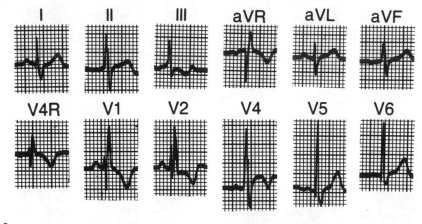

FIG 5—6.
Tracing from a 4-year-old girl with secundum type of atrial septal defect.

In Figure 5—6, all the voltages are within normal limits. The R/S ratio in V2 is abnormal, being greater than the ULN for the patient's age (1.5), indicating abnormally strong anterior force suggestive of RVH. On closer inspection there is some terminal slurring of the QRS complex which is directed anteriorly and rightward (slurred R′ in V4R, V1, and aVR, and slurred S in I, V5, and V6). QRS duration (0.09 second) is slightly beyond the ULN (0.08 second). The rsR′ pattern is present in V1. The T vector is normal. The diagnosis of RBBB, rather than RVH, is justified in this case.

Interpretation: RBBB.

LEFT BUNDLE BRANCH BLOCK (LBBB)

When the left bundle branch is interrupted, there is an abnormality of septal depolarization. The septal depolarization is normally initiated by fibers of the left bundle branch and is in the direction of left to right. Instead, the septal depolarization proceeds leftward from the RV in LBBB (labeled "1" in Fig 5–7), resulting in the loss of q waves in the LPLs. The RV depolarization is normal ("2" in Fig 5–7). The LV is depolarized through the ventricular myocardium at a much slower rate ("3" in the Fig 5–7), producing prolongation of QRS duration. Therefore, in LBBB, abnormalities are found not only in the terminal phase but in the initial phase of ventricular depolarization, affecting the entire QRS complex. The wide QRS complex is directed to the *left* and *posteriorly,* with resulting slurred R in the LPLs and slurred S in the RPLs (see Fig 5–7). Because of asynchrony of depolarization of the two ventricles as in RBBB, the QRS voltages may be abnormal, but hypertrophy should not be inferred. Since all phases of normal activation are altered, myocardial infarction cannot be diagnosed (see Chap. 6).

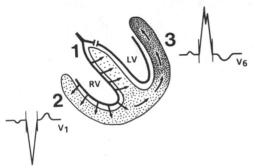

FIG 5–7.
Sequence of ventricular depolarization in LBBB. Note that the septal depolarization proceeds in direction opposite of normal, producing a Q wave in V1 but not in V6. The wide QRS complex is directed leftward and posteriorly, producing wide S in V1 and wide R in V6.

Criteria for LBBB (Summary)

1. Left axis deviation for the patient's age (see Figs 3–2 and 3–3).
2. QRS duration longer than the ULN for the patient's age (see Table 3–2).
3. Loss of Q waves in I, V5, and V6.
4. The slurred QRS complex is directed to the left and posteriorly (see Fig 3–3).
   a. Slurred and wide R waves in I, aVL, V5, and V6.
   b. Wide S waves in V1 and V2.
5. ST depression and T wave inversion in V4 through V6 are common.
6. QRS voltages may be greater than normal because of the asynchrony of depolarization of each ventricle. One should not make a diagnosis of ventricular hypertrophy when LBBB is present.

Although LBBB is relatively common in adults in association with ischemic and hypertensive heart disease, it is extremely rare in children. However, for the sake of completeness and comparison with RBBB, an example of LBBB from an elderly person is presented (Fig 5–8).

Example (Fig 5–8)

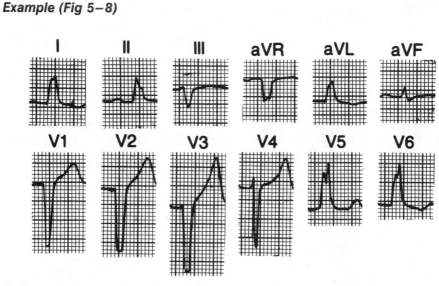

FIG 5–8.
Tracing from a 76-year-old man with complaints of chest pain and hypertension.

HEMIBLOCKS OR FASCICULAR BLOCKS

We have described the LBBB as if there were only one left bundle branch, but in fact the left bundle branch consists of three divisions or fascicles: (1) septal; (2) anterior-superior; and (3) posterior-inferior. When viewed in the frontal projection, the anterior division looks higher than the posterior division (Fig 5–9). In children only the anterior fascicle is of clinical significance. When delay or block occurs in these fascicles, hemiblock or fascicular block is diagnosed. Some authorities object to the term *hemiblock* since there are more than two fascicles.

When the anterior division is blocked, the superior anterior portion of the LV will be depolarized last and the QRS vector will be directed supero-anteriorly, producing a marked left axis deviation (LAD) (less than −30 degrees) on the hexaxial reference system. When the posterior division is blocked, the LV depolarization is directed inferiorly and to the right, producing right axis deviation (RAD). Since the posterior fascicle branches immediately into a wide network, complete interruption is unlikely, particularly in children. Anterior fascicular block, in contrast, is characteristic of certain congenital heart defects (endocardial cushion defect, tricuspid atresia) in children. Left anterior hemiblock (or fascicular block) is often referred to as superior QRS axis in the pediatric literature. There is usually no prolongation of the QRS duration in hemiblocks because the Purkinje fibers in the LV are richly confluent.

Left anterior hemiblock (superior QRS axis) is manifested by (1) marked LAD (−30 to −90 degrees) and (2) little or no prolongation of QRS duration. It is a characteristic finding in children with endocardial cushion defect or tricuspid atresia (see Figs 9–5 and 9–11). In adults it is due to myocardial infarction or fibrosis resulting from coronary artery disease or chronic left heart failure.

Left posterior hemiblock is manifested by marked RAD and normal QRS duration. It is extremely rare in children.

As can be seen in Figure 5–9, there are four major fascicles or divisions of the ventricular conduction system. *Bifascicular block* indicates blockage of any two fascicles. In children the combination of RBBB and left anterior hemiblock is frequently seen in the primum type of atrial septal defect (partial endocardial cushion defect). This combination of bifascicular block (RBBB plus left anterior hemiblock) is also seen postoperatively in children after repair of tetralogy of Fallot; whether it is ominous then or not is uncertain. In adults the combined abnormality may be acquired during an acute myocardial infarction and is cause for alarm in

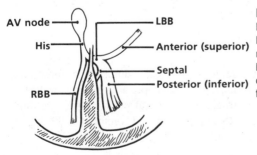

FIG 5–9.
Diagram of right and left bundle branches. Note that the right bundle branch *(RBB)* remains as a single fascicle, while the left bundle branch *(LBB)* subdivides into three divisions: *septal, anterior,* and *posterior* fascicles.

cases of coronary artery disease. This may be seen from Figure 5–9; an ischemic lesion that involves two fascicles (bifascicular block) is anatomically very close to involving all of the fascicles and/or the bundle of His, producing complete heart block (see Chap. 7). Complete heart block, acutely acquired, could be fatal in an older patient and warrants consideration of prophylactic pacemaker therapy in patients with acutely acquired bifascicular block.

INTRAVENTRICULAR BLOCK

A prolonged QRS duration (beyond the ULN) may occur without the characteristic changes of either RBBB or LBBB because of a diffuse conduction delay throughout the ventricles rather than a block in one of the bundle branches. The QRS is slurred throughout the QRS complex rather than just terminal or initial slurring (Figs 5–1 and 5–10). This type of block is associated with metabolic disorders, diffuse myocardial disease, severe hypoxia, or drug toxicity (quinidine, procainamide, etc.).

Example (Fig 5–10)

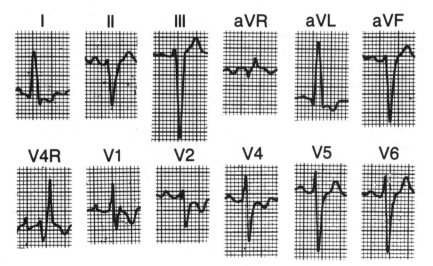

FIG 5–10.
Tracing from a 15-year-old girl with systemic lupus erythematosus.

In Figure 5–10, the mean QRS axis is −60 degrees. The QRS duration is abnormally prolonged (0.15 second). The maximal QRS duration in normal people at this age is 0.10 second (see Table 3–2). The slurring is not confined to either the initial portion or the terminal portion of the QRS complex; it is throughout the QRS complex. The T vector is +90 degrees in the frontal plane, with a wide QRS-T angle (130 degrees).

Interpretation: Intraventricular block.

Rarely, prolongation of the QRS duration is seen in ventricular hypertrophy, even without conduction delays. Increased muscle mass in ventricular hypertrophy increases the total time for ventricular depolarization in an incremental fashion, resulting in a prolonged QRS. Thus, a ventricular conduction disturbance (with a wide QRS duration) alone can increase QRS voltages, and ventricular hypertrophy (with increased QRS voltages) can also manifest with a wide QRS duration. Because of this overlap, differentiation between ventricular conduction disturbances and ventricular hypertrophy is not always possible, when one deals with abnormally wide *and* abnormally tall (or deep) QRS complexes. The following guidelines may help in interpreting wide and tall QRS complexes.

1. When there is an initial slurring ("delta" wave) with increased QRS duration and QRS voltages, the large QRS complexes are due to preexcitation (WPW syndrome), not due to ventricular hypertrophy.

2. When there is a clear terminal slurring with increased QRS duration and voltages, the diagnosis of RBBB is justified. However, rarely a BBB pattern with slightly increased QRS duration may result from ventricular hypertrophy (Fig 9–18 is an example).

3. When the QRS duration is prolonged throughout, without initial or terminal slurring, large QRS voltages are more often secondary to ventricular hypertrophy than conduction delay. Intraventricular blocks are less frequently associated with large QRS voltages than with RBBB.

IMPLANTED VENTRICULAR PACEMAKER

A patient with complete heart block may require an artificial pacemaker implanted in the endocardium or epicardium of a ventricle. The ventricle in which the pacemaker is implanted will be depolarized first, followed by the other ventricle through myocardial transmission. Therefore, the QRS duration will be prolonged and the QRS complex will resemble that of right or left BBB, depending upon the site of implantation. For example, a pacemaker implanted in the LV will produce QRS complexes that resemble RBBB (Fig 5–11). The same approach may be applied to identify the site of focus of premature ventricular contractions (PVCs); if the abnormal focus is in the LV, a RBBB pattern will be produced. If the abnormal focus is in the RV, the PVC will resemble the QRS complex of LBBB.

Example (Fig 5–11)

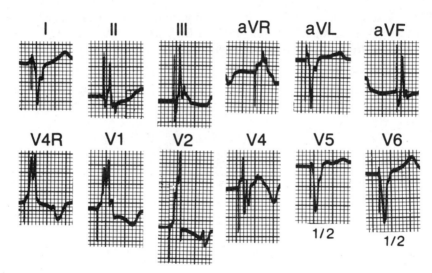

FIG 5–11.
Tracing from a 7-year-old girl with congenital heart block who received a fixed-rate ventricular pacemaker because of fainting spells. The pacemaker was implanted in the LV epicardium. The QRS morphology resembles that of RBBB, with slurred S waves in leads I, V5, and V6, and slurred R waves in the right precordial leads.

In Figure 5–11, each QRS complex is preceded by a sharp pacemaker spike. QRS complexes are abnormally long in duration (about 0.12 second) and resemble those of RBBB, i.e., deep, prolonged S waves in I, V5, and V6, and slurred R waves in aVR and the RPLs. The T vector is, in general, opposite to the QRS vector. These findings suggest the LV as the implantation site. There are P waves in random relationship to the QRS complexes seen in aVR, V4R, and V2 (complete heart block, and fixed rate ventricular pacing). The duration and amplitude of the P waves are abnormally increased.

Interpretation: Fixed rate ventricular pacemaker implanted in the LV, complete heart block, and probable combined atrial hypertrophy.

Artificial Cardiac Pacemakers

Although detailed discussion of pacemaker is beyond the scope of this book, ECG patterns of different types of artificial pacemakers will be presented. Depending on the position and number of the pacemaker spikes, the artificial pacemaker may be classified as follows:

Ventricular Pacemakers (Ventricular Sensing and Pacing)

This mode of pacing is recognized by vertical pacemaker spikes that initiate ventricular depolarization with wide QRS complexes (Figs 5–11 and 5–12,A). The electronic spike has no fixed relationship with atrial activity, and there is usually no P wave in front of the spike, except by coincidence. The pacemaker rate may be fixed (see Fig 5–12,A) or it may be on a demand (or standby) mode. In a *fixed-rate* ventricular pacemaker the electronic spikes come at regular intervals, and the rate is set by the manufacturer or may be programmable. In *demand* (or *standby*) mode, the pacemaker fires only after a long pause between the patient's own ventricular beats or when the patient's spontaneous rate drops below the programmed rate. If there is an early R wave, the demand pacemaker is inhibited. The length of the pause that triggers the pacemaker is preset or programmable.

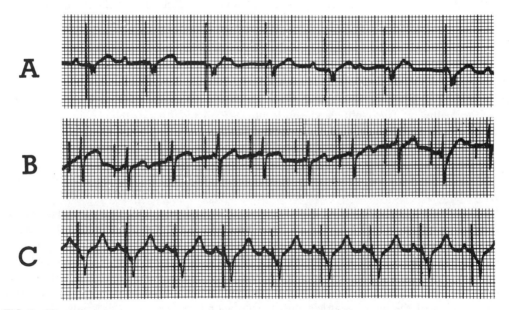

FIG 5–12.
Examples of some artificial pacemakers. **A,** fixed-rate ventricular pacemaker. Note the regular rate of the electronic spikes with no relationship to the P waves. The electronic spikes are large and are followed by relatively wide and small-voltage QRS complexes. **B,** atrial pacemaker. This tracing is from a 2-year-old child in whom extreme, symptomatic sinus bradycardia developed following surgical repair for transposition of the great arteries. There is an atrial complex following the atrial electronic spike. The QRS complex is of normal duration because the AV nodal conduction is normal. **C,** P-wave triggered ventricular pacemaker. This tracing is from a child in whom surgically induced complete heart block developed following repair of tetralogy of Fallot. The patient's own P wave triggers QRS complexes through a ventricular pacemaker; resulting in wide QRS complexes.

Atrial Pacemaker (Atrial Sensing and Pacing)

The atrial pacemaker is recognized by a pacemaker spike followed by an atrial complex; when there is normal AV conduction, a QRS complex of normal duration will follow (Fig 5–12,B). The atrial pacemaker usually operates in the demand mode, and the rate is fixed but programmable. When there is high-degree or complete AV block in addition to sinus node dysfunction with sinus bradycardia, a ventricular pacemaker may also be required (AV sequential pacemaker). The AV sequential pacemaker is recognized by two sets of electronic spikes: one before the P wave and another before the wide QRS complex. Although this type of pacing is more physiologic than the ventricular sensing and pacing type, the rate cannot increase with activity.

P-Wave–Triggered Ventricular Pacemaker (Atrial Sensing, Ventricular Pacing)

This pacemaker may be recognized by pacemaker spikes that follow the patient's own P waves, at regular PR intervals, and with wide QRS complexes (Fig 5–12,C). The patient's own P waves are sensed, which triggers a ventricular pacemaker after an electronically preset PR interval. This type of pacemaker is most physiologic and indicated when there is an AV block but the sinus mechanism is normal. The advantages of this type of pacemaker are that (1) the heart rate varies with physiologic needs, and (2) the atrial contraction contributes to ventricular filling and improves cardiac output.

PREEXCITATION

Preexcitation is defined as accelerated atrioventricular conduction to one ventricle through an accessory pathway. The Wolff-Parkinson-White (WPW) syndrome is the classic form of preexcitation, with episodes of AV reentry tachycardia.

Anomalous AV Conduction (Wolff-Parkinson-White Syndrome)

The WPW syndrome results from an anomalous conduction pathway (Kent bundle) between the atrium and the ventricle (either side), bypassing the AV node. Without the normal delay in the AV conduction the ventricle that is connected to the anomalous bundle gets depolarized prematurely at a slower rate, through the ventricular myocardium (*1a* in Fig 5–13), producing the delta wave (initial slurring) and short PR interval. Remember that the latter part of the PR interval (PQ segment) represents the delay in the AV node, and absence of the normal delay will shorten this segment. After the normal delay in the AV node but before completion of depolarization of the entire ventricle through the anomalous pathway, the remainder of the ventricles is depolarized in normal fashion through the Purkinje system (see *1* and *2* in Fig 5–13). Because of the asynchrony in depolarization of both ventricles, potentials for each ventricle may become exaggerated.

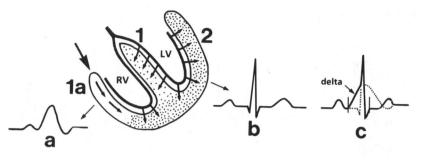

FIG 5–13.
Sequence of ventricular depolarization in the WPW syndrome and the mechanism for generation of abnormal QRS complex.

If the entire ventricle is depolarized through the abnormal pathway *(1a)*, the ventricular complex will be wide, as shown in *"a"* in Figure 5–13, because of the slow conduction velocity through the ventricular myocardium. However, before completion of depolarization of the entire ventricle, normal antegrade conduction occurs *(1* and *2)*, with normal depolarization of the remainder of the ventricle *(b)*. The end result is superimposition of *"a* and *b,"* resulting in the typical P-QRS complex of the WPW syndrome *(c)*. In this condition, the sum of PR interval and QRS duration is unaltered. Asynchronous excitation and lack of normal cancellation of opposing forces invalidates voltage criteria for ventricular hypertrophy. (Fig 5–15 illustrates schematically the abnormal Kent bundle which bypasses the AV node.)

Criteria for WPW Syndrome

1. Short PR interval, less than the lower limits of normal (LLN) for the patient's age. The LLN according to age is as follows:

    Lower Limit of Normal PR Interval:

Less than 3 years	0.08 second
3–16 years	0.10 second
More than 16 years	0.12 second

2. Delta wave (initial slurring of the QRS complex).
3. Wide QRS duration (beyond the ULN).

Example (Fig 5–14)

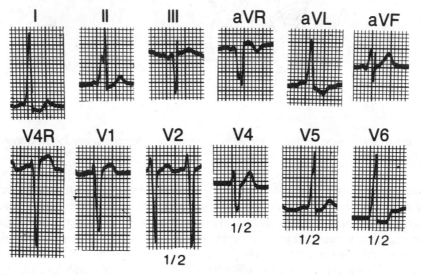

FIG 5–14.
Tracing from a 6-month-old infant with possible glycogen storage disease. There was no history of paroxysmal tachycardia.

In Figure 5–14, the QRS axis is 0 degrees. The QRS duration is increased to 0.10 second (ULN = 0.06). The PR interval is short (0.07). There are delta waves in the initial portion of the QRS complex, best seen in I, aVL, and V5. Since the vector of the delta wave is leftward, as well as only slightly anterior, the preexcitation probably occurs in the right ventricle. The leftward and posterior QRS voltages are abnormally large, but with preexcitation, the diagnosis of LVH cannot be made.

Interpretation: WPW type preexcitation.

Classification

Classification into types A and B has been used for some time. However, there is an infinite number of possible sites where the bundle of Kent can be found around the mitral or tricuspid valves or through the ventricular septum. Therefore, this classification into A and B types has only historical significance.

Clinical Significance

The WPW syndrome has important clinical significance.

1. Patients with the WPW syndrome are prone to attacks of supraventricular tachycardia (SVT) of the reciprocating or reentry type (see Chap. 7). During the attacks, however, the QRS complex is not usually abnormal because preexcitation does not occur during tachycardias. The bypass bundle is involved in retrograde conduction, completing the reentry pathway (see Chap. 7 for reentry).

2. The WPW syndrome may mimic other ECG abnormalities, such as RVH, LVH, BBB, or myocardial disorders and result in erroneous diagnosis.

3. The WPW syndrome may accompany congenital heart disease. Ebstein's anomaly is the most common defect to be associated with this syndrome, and patients with glycogen storage disease frequently demonstrate preexcitation (see Fig 5–14). Other lesions such as tetralogy of Fallot, L-transposition of the great arteries, and the primum type of atrial septal defect have also been reported to be associated with this syndrome, but not often.

Enhanced AV Conduction (Lown-Ganong-Levine Syndrome)

Lown-Ganong-Levine (LGL) syndrome is characterized by short PR and normal QRS duration in patients with episodes of supraventricular tachycardia. In these patients the upper AV node is bypassed (via James fibers), producing a short PR interval, but the ventricles are depolarized normally through the His-Purkinje system (Fig 5–15). These bypass fibers also create the necessary circuit for reentry tachycardia (see Chap. 7 for reentry). Alternatively, enhanced AV conduction could occur in the fast pathway in dual pathway AV nodes, which are a common substrate of SVT.

Anomalous Nodoventricular Connection (Mahaim Fibers)

This is characterized by normal PR interval and long QRS duration with delta wave. An accessory fiber (Mahaim fiber) between the AV node and one of the ventricles, usually the right ventricle, produces the delta wave and long QRS duration. The normal delay in conduction in the AV node accounts for the relatively normal PR interval (see Fig 5–15), although the PR may be short.

Multiple Anomalous Connections.—Rarely, more than one accessory fiber may be present. These may be difficult to detect without elimination of the first set of fibers, pharmacologically or surgically.

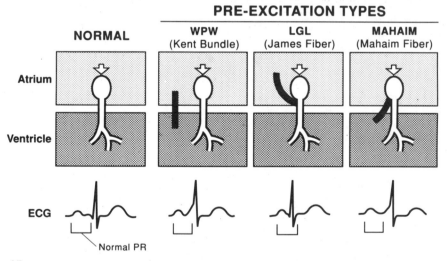

PRE-EXCITATION TYPES

FIG 5–15.
Schematic diagram of accessory pathways and the electrocardiogram in preexcitation. In the normal person, the only way the atrial impulse *(open arrow)* reaches the ventricle is through AV node and the bundle of His. In preexcitation, abnormal pathways partially bypass the normal conduction system. The bundle of Kent is responsible for the majority of cases of WPW syndrome. James fibers bypass the upper AV node in LGL syndrome. In Mahaim-type preexcitation, Mahaim fibers bypass the bundle of His and "short-circuit" into the right ventricle.

REVIEW QUESTIONS

Answer the following four questions based on the tracing from a 3-year-old child shown in Figure 5–16.

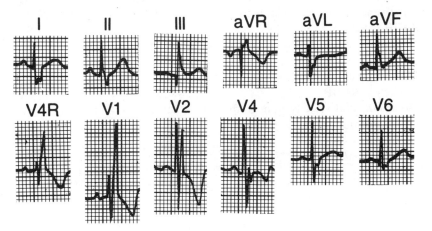

FIG 5–16.

1. The QRS duration is:
    a. Normal for age
    b. Prolonged for age
    c. Too short for age
2. The slurring is in:
    a. The initial portion of the QRS complex
    b. The terminal portion
    c. Throughout the QRS complex
3. The slurring is directed:
    a. Rightward only
    b. Rightward and anteriorly
    c. Leftward and posteriorly
    d. Posteriorly
4. Based on the above, which of the following is present?
    a. RBBB
    b. LBBB
    c. Intraventricular block
    d. WPW syndrome
5. Which of the following does *not* prolong the QRS duration?
    a. Implanted ventricular pacemaker
    b. RBBB
    c. WPW syndrome
    d. Left anterior hemiblock
6. Short PR intervals may be seen in:
    a. First-degree AV block
    b. Complete heart block
    c. Digitalis toxicity
    d. Hyperkalemia
    e. None of the above

Answer the following questions either "true" or "false."

7. The Q wave is produced primarily by the depolarization of the ventricular septum.   True   False
8. RBBB is almost always associated with right axis deviation.   True   False
9. If the ventricular pacemaker is implanted in the left ventricle, an RBBB pattern is produced.   True   False
10. The QRS duration of 0.08 second is abnormally long in a new-born infant, although it is normal in an adult.   True   False
11. The most common form of ventricular conduction disturbance in children is RBBB.   True   False
12. The conduction velocity through the ventricular myocardium is as fast as that through the His-Purkinje system.   True   False

Answers may be found on pages 238 and 239.

CHAPTER 6

Changes in ST Segment
and T Wave

In the electrocardiograms (ECGs) of adults, shifts of the ST segment and T wave changes are common as a result of a high incidence of ischemic heart disease, myocardial infarction, bundle branch blocks, and other myocardial disorders. In pediatric ECGs, however, ST and T changes are relatively infrequent because of a low incidence of myocardial disorders.

NONPATHOLOGIC ST SEGMENT SHIFT

Not all ST segment shifts are abnormal. Slight shift is common in normal children. Elevation or depression up to 1 mm in the limb leads and up to 2 mm in the precordial leads are within normal limits. Two important types of nonpathologic ST segment shifts seen in pediatric patients are J-depression and early repolarization. These nonpathologic shifts are not accompanied by T wave changes.

J-Depression

J-depression is a shift of the junction between the QRS and the ST segment (J-point) without sustained ST segment depression (Fig 6–1,A). The T waves are not altered.

Early Repolarization

In this condition, all leads with an upright T wave have elevated ST segments and leads with negative T waves have depressed ST segments (Fig 6–2). This is associated with a relatively

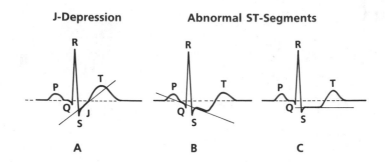

FIG 6–1.
Nonpathologic (nonischemic) and pathologic (ischemic) ST and T changes. **A,** characteristic nonischemic ST segment alteration called J-depression; note that the ST slope is upward. **B,** and **C,** examples of ischemic or pathologic ST segment alterations; note that there is a downward slope of the ST segment **(B)** or the horizontal segment is sustained **(C).**

tall T wave. The T vector remains normal. This ST segment shift is stable and does not evolve gradually as it does in acute pericarditis (discussed later), an important differential point. In some instances this phenomenon may be produced by a poor frequency response of the ECG recorder in the presence of tachycardia. In its true form, the ST segment shift is thought to represent early repolarization of some areas of the ventricular myocardium.

Example of Early Repolarization (Fig 6–2)

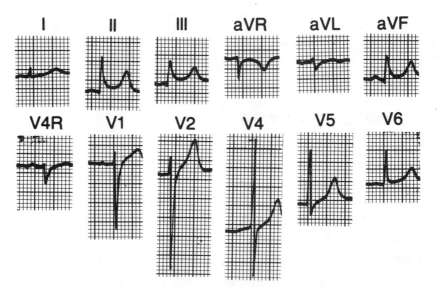

FIG 6–2.
Tracing from a healthy 16-year-old boy that exhibits early repolarization.

In Figure 6–2, the QRS axis is +80 degrees. The T axis is also about +60 degrees. The J point is not clearly defined, and therefore, accurate determination of the QRS duration is difficult, but appears to be within normal limits. The ST segment is shifted toward the direction of the T wave, most marked in leads II, III, and aVF. The QRS voltages are normal for age. No pathologic Q wave is present.

Interpretation: Early repolarization.

PATHOLOGIC ST-T CHANGES

Abnormal shifts of the ST segment are often accompanied by T wave changes. An abnormal ST segment shift assumes one of the following two forms (see Fig 6–1):

1. Downward slanting followed by diphasic or inverted T wave (Fig 6–1,B), or
2. Straight or horizontal ST segment sustained for over 0.08 second (Fig 6–1,C).

Conditions that produce abnormal ST segment and T wave changes in children are:

1. LVH or RVH with "strain."
2. Digitalis effect.
3. Pericarditis, including postoperative state.
4. Myocarditis.
5. Myocardial ischemia.
6. Myocardial infarction.
7. Electrolyte disturbances; hypokalemia and hyperkalemia.

These conditions will be discussed in the pages that follow.

Other conditions that are associated with T wave changes with or without ST segment shift include right and left bundle branch blocks, preexcitation (WPW syndrome), premature ventricular contractions, and paroxysmal tachycardias. These conditions, however, will not be discussed in this chapter (see Chapters 5 and 7).

LVH or RVH With "Strain"

The ST shift seen in severe ventricular hypertrophy with "strain" has the same orientation as the T vector, which is generally away from the hypertrophied ventricle. This results in:

1. ST segment depression and sharply inverted T wave in leads that represent the left or right ventricle (see Fig 6–3,A), and
2. Wide QRS-T angle with the T vector outside the normal quadrant (see Fig 4–7).

See Chapter 4, hypertrophy, for further details.

FIG 6–3.

ST-T changes in ventricular hypertrophy with "strain" and digitalis effect. **A,** ST segment and T wave are shifted opposite to the direction of the major QRS deflection in leads representing the respective hypertrophied ventricle. QRS-T angle is wide (greater than 90 degrees) with the T vector outside the normal quadrant. **B,** ST segment is shifted opposite to the direction of the major QRS deflection. QT interval is shortened. T wave is either small or diphasic but T vector remains in the normal quadrant, unless it was abnormal prior to digitalization.

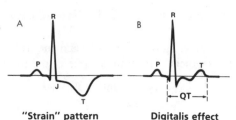

"Strain" pattern   Digitalis effect

Digitalis Effect

The ECG alterations of digitalis effect—in contrast to toxicity—are confined to ventricular repolarization and consist of the following (see Fig 6–3,B):

1. Shortening of corrected QT interval (QTc) is the earliest sign.
2. Depression of terminal portion of ST segment, producing sagging ST segment.
3. Diminished magnitude of T wave but with no change in the T vector, at least at rest. (The T vector may change with exercise.) Therefore, the QRS-T angle is normal. An abnormally wide QRS-T angle in a patient receiving digitalis suggests that an abnormality was present before digitalization. (A control ECG before digitalization is mandatory.)

Pericarditis

The ECG changes seen in pericarditis are the result of subepicardial myocardial damage and/or pericardial effusion.

1. Subepicardial myocardial damage produces the following time-dependent changes in the ST segment and T wave (Fig 6–4):
   a. Elevation of ST segment in many limb and precordial leads, particularly those representing the LV.
   b. Within two to three days the ST segment returns close to normal. The T wave is small but still upright. It is difficult to detect the abnormality at this stage.
   c. Two to four weeks after the onset, T waves become sharply inverted and there is an isoelectric ST segment. This change may persist one to two months.
2. Pericardial effusion may result in low QRS voltages in many leads. Low voltages are said to be present when the amplitude of the QRS complexes in every one of the limb leads is 5 mm or less. The low voltage is due to short-circuiting of the electrical forces by the surrounding fluid.

Acute myocardial infarction produces ECG findings similar to those of pericarditis. The main differences are that in acute myocardial infarction the changes are more localized, ST segment and T wave changes occur simultaneously, and pathologic Q waves appear (see following section on myocardial infarction).

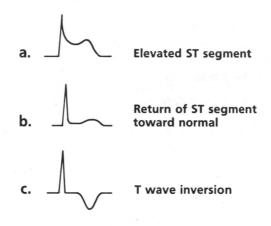

a.   Elevated ST segment

b.   Return of ST segment toward normal

c.   T wave inversion

FIG 6–4.
Time-dependent changes of ST segment and T wave in pericarditis.

Example (Fig 6–5)

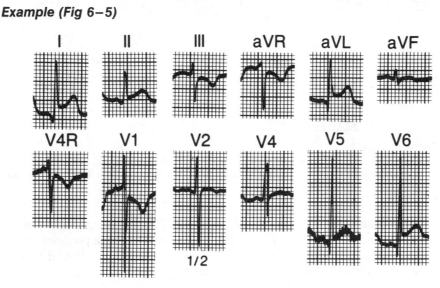

FIG 6–5.
Tracing from a 10-year-old boy with Duchenne's muscular dystrophy and clinical findings of acute pericarditis. The heart rate was 140 beats per minute.

In Figure 6–5, the rhythm is sinus. The QRS axis is +10 degrees, which is relatively leftward for the patient's age, and the T axis is 0 degrees. The QRS amplitudes and the R/S ratios are all within normal limits, although the R wave in V6 is at the ULN (24 mm). The relatively tall R in V6 and leftward QRS axis raise the possibility of mild LVH. The QRS amplitude is normal in the limb leads. The most remarkable abnormality is the ST segment elevation seen in many leads that represent the LV (I, II, aVL, V5, V6, etc.). The QRS voltages are not abnormally low. The uneven baseline seen in V5 is an artifact. Note one-half standardization in V2.

Interpretation: ST segment shift compatible with acute pericarditis, and possible LVH.

Myocarditis

Electrocardiographic findings of myocarditis (rheumatic or viral) are relatively nonspecific and may include changes in all phases of the cardiac cycle, even arrhythmias or ectopic beats. One or more of the following changes are seen in myocarditis:

1. Delayed AV conduction (first-degree AV block).
2. Prolongation of QTc.
3. Decreased amplitude of the T wave.
4. Low QRS amplitude, i.e., 5 mm or less in all six limb leads (Fig 6–6).
5. Arrhythmias or ectopic beats.

Example (Fig 6–6)

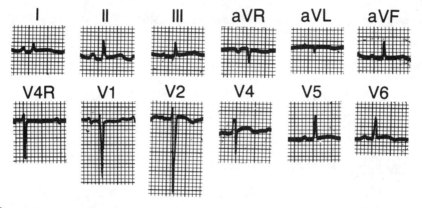

FIG 6–6.
Tracing from a 14-month-old infant with a clinical diagnosis of viral myocarditis. The heart rate was 140 beats per minute.

In Figure 6–6, the rhythm is sinus. The PR interval is 0.12 and the QRS duration is 0.05, both within normal limits. The QT interval is 0.28, which is at the upper limits of normal (ULN) for the heart rate. The T waves are low in amplitude throughout. The QRS amplitude is low also, being less than 5 mm in every one of the limb leads.

Interpretation: Low-voltage QRS complexes and T waves, suggestive of pancarditis.

Myocardial Infarction

Although myocardial infarction is rare in pediatric cases, a brief discussion will be included for the sake of completeness.

In the early phase of acute myocardial infarction, three electrically distinct zones are present: the zone of *necrosis* (center) is surrounded by a zone of *injury,* which in turn is surrounded by a zone of *ischemia* (Fig 6–7). No depolarization occurs in the necrotic area; leads facing the necrotic area will record depolarization from live myocardium *away* from the electrode, producing the pathologic Q wave. A lead facing the area of injury will record an ST vector shift *toward* the lead, producing ST segment elevation. (The injured cells are partially depolarized and actually create a depression of the entire baseline [TP and PQ segments] with the exception of the ST segment; owing to the recording characteristics of ECG machines, this

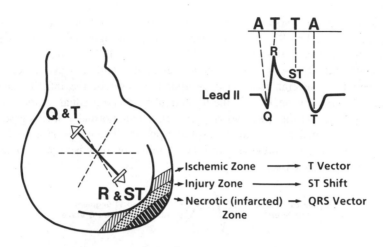

FIG 6–7.

Correlation between pathology and ECG changes in acute myocardial infarction. A lead (II in this case) oriented toward the zone of necrosis, injury, and ischemia records a pathologic Q wave, an elevated ST segment, and an inverted T wave, respectively. An acronym, ATTA, can be employed to remember that the ECG shows the initial QRS vector (Q wave) moving away from the area of infarction, the terminal QRS vector moving *toward* it, the ST segment shift *toward* it and the T wave change *away* from it. (Modified from a drawing by Constant J: *Learning Electrocardiography*. Boston, Little Brown & Co, 1973.)

appears as an ST elevation.) The leads facing the ischemic area record the T vector going *away* from the area (see Fig 6–7). Thus, a lead facing the area of infarct will record all three patterns, including a pathologic Q wave (wide and deep), ST segment elevation, and T wave inversion. The *pathologic Q waves* of myocardial infarction are of longer duration (at least 0.03 second and usually 0.04 second) and of greater amplitude than normal (see Chap. 3 for normal amplitude of Q waves). Often the terminal portion of the QRS complex is opposite to the Q wave (peri-infarction block).

The term *peri-infarction block* is used to describe the terminal QRS vector that is slightly prolonged and is directed toward an infarct. This phenomenon occurs almost exclusively in anterolateral and inferior infarctions. An infarct involving one of the fascicles may make the area distal to the infarct depolarize later than the intact area of the myocardium. This will result in the terminal QRS vector being directed toward the area of infarct. For example, the anterolateral myocardial infarction may involve the anterosuperior fascicle (see Fig 5–9) with resulting delayed depolarization of the anterolateral aspect of the left ventricle. It is also believed that depolarization takes longer to travel through the area around the infarct, producing delayed activation of the tissue around the infarction. Requirements for peri-infarction block consist of a pathologic Q wave and slight terminal slurring directed opposite to the Q wave.

The ECG findings of myocardial infarction are time-dependent. The short-lived hyperacute phase, characterized by ST segment elevation and pathologic Q wave, is seen during the first few hours after the infarction (Fig 6–8). More common ECG findings of myocardial infarction are abnormal Q waves, ST segment elevations, and T wave inversions. These changes are seen from several hours to days after the onset of the infarct (early evolving phase). During the first few weeks after the infarction there is a gradual return of the elevated ST segment toward the baseline (late evolving phase). The abnormal T waves gradually return to a normal or near-normal configuration (resolving phase). Therefore, in a stabilized old infarction the only evidence of a previous myocardial infarction may be a pathologic Q wave in leads oriented to the infarcted scar.

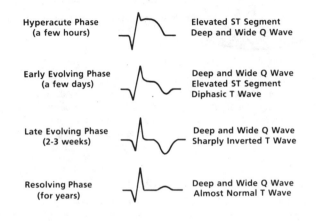

Hyperacute Phase (a few hours) — Elevated ST Segment / Deep and Wide Q Wave

Early Evolving Phase (a few days) — Deep and Wide Q Wave / Elevated ST Segment / Diphasic T Wave

Late Evolving Phase (2-3 weeks) — Deep and Wide Q Wave / Sharply Inverted T Wave

Resolving Phase (for years) — Deep and Wide Q Wave / Almost Normal T Wave

FIG 6–8.
Sequential changes of ST segment and T wave in myocardial infarction.

Most myocardial infarctions are located in the left ventricular free wall and ventricular septum. The ventricular septum is considered as the anterior wall of the left ventricle in the adult, in whom the right ventricle is relatively silent. The characteristic time-dependent ECG findings of myocardial infarction (see Fig 6–8) are best seen in the leads, the positive terminals of which are closest to the area of infarction. Figure 6–9 illustrates the common locations of infarctions and the limb and/or precordial leads that demonstrate the characteristic ECG findings for each location (see also Table 6–1). Peri-infarction blocks are commonly seen in anterolateral and inferior (diaphragmatic) infarctions. For example, a few days after the onset of a lateral myocardial infarction, the characteristic ECG findings (pathologic Q waves, ST segment elevation, T wave inversion, and peri-infarction block) will be best seen in leads I, aVL, V5, and V6. The limb leads usually do not show evidence of infarction in the strictly posterior or anterior wall, since the frontal plane leads do not represent the anteroposterior relationship. For similar reasons, the strictly inferior infarction will not show up in the horizontal plane or precordial leads.

Occasionally the ST shift will not be consistent with the scheme just presented in that the vector for the ST shift will be away from the infarct. This is attributable to a subendocardial ischemia as opposed to the epicardial infarction diagrammed in Figure 6–7.

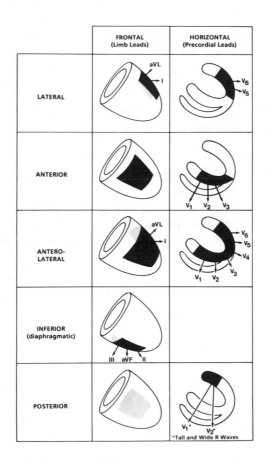

FIG 6–9.
Schematic drawing of the location of myocardial infarction and ECG leads that are expected to show findings of myocardial infarction (see Table 6–1, below).

TABLE 6–1.

Leads Showing Abnormal ECG Findings in
Myocardial Infarction

	Limb Leads	Precordial Leads
Lateral	I, aVL	V5, V6
Anterior		V1, V2, V3
Anterolateral	I, aVL	V2–V6
Diaphragmatic	II, III, aVF	
Posterior		V1–V3*

*None of the leads is oriented toward the posterior surface of
the heart. Therefore, in posterior infarction, changes that
would have been present in the posterior surface leads will
be seen in the anterior leads as a mirror image, e.g., tall and
slightly wide R waves in V1 and V2, comparable to abnormal
Q waves, and tall and wide, symmetric T waves in V1 and
V2.

Non-Q Wave Myocardial Infarction.—In the past an acute myocardial infarction in which Q waves failed to develop on the ECG was referred to as a "subendocardial" or "non-transmural" myocardial infarction with depressed, rather than elevated, ST segments. However, the presence or absence of Q waves on the ECG does not always correlate with pathological findings of transmural or non-transmural infarction. True subendocardial myocardial infarction is seen with ST-segment depression and/or T wave changes in only 50% of the cases. The diagnosis of non-transmural infarction rests more on the combination of clinical findings and the elevation of serum enzymes than the ECG.

In children, a myocardial infarction pattern may be seen in association with anomalous left coronary artery arising from the pulmonary artery (Fig 6–10), coronary artery embolization from bacterial endocarditis or diagnostic procedures performed on the left side of the heart, inadvertent surgical interruption of the coronary artery, endocardial fibroelastosis, and arteritis (mucocutaneous lymph node syndrome of Kawasaki). It may rarely be seen following difficult cases of the Jatene operation (arterial switch operation) for transposition of the great arteries, due to a kink in the transposed coronary arteries.

Example (Fig 6–10)

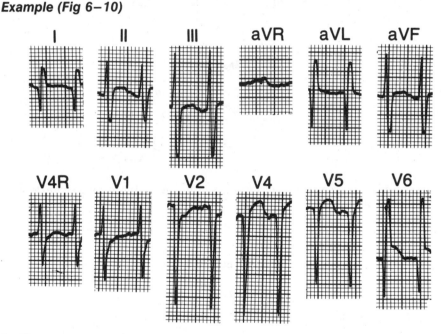

FIG 6–10.
Tracing from a 2-month-old male infant who has anomalous origin of the left coronary artery from the pulmonary artery.

In Figure 6–10, the most impressive finding is the presence of deep and wide (0.04 second) Q waves in leads I, aVL, and V6. A QS pattern is present in V2 through V5. Abnormal findings seen in leads I and aVL, and in precordial leads V2 through V6 are consistent with antero-lateral myocardial infarction. The QRSi is +120 degrees (away from the infarcted area). The terminal portion of the QRS complex is slightly prolonged and the QRSt is −65 degrees (toward the infarct). This suggests peri-infarction block. ST segment elevation is present in a few limb leads and in the left precordial leads. The P wave is partially hidden in the terminal portion of the T wave.

Interpretation: Acute anterolateral myocardial infarction.

Electrolyte Disturbances

Two important serum electrolytes that produce ECG changes are calcium (Ca) and potassium (K). Changes in concentrations of other serum electrolytes such as sodium or magnesium have no specific effects on the ECG. Although hypocalcemia and hypercalcemia do not produce ST segment shift, they will be discussed in this chapter since they change the relative position of the T wave.

    1. Hypocalcemia.—The calcium ion is mainly concerned with phase 2 of the action potential and affects only the duration of the ST segment. Hypocalcemia prolongs the ST segment with resulting prolongation of QTc; however, it does not alter the duration or vector of the T wave. The ST segment remains isoelectric. The T wave is simply delayed, not actually widened (Fig 6–11).

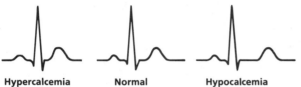

Hypercalcemia   **Normal**   **Hypocalcemia**

FIG 6–11.
ECG findings of hypercalcemia and hypocalcemia. Hypercalcemia shortens and hypocalcemia lengthens the ST segment. The T wave is not altered.

    2. Hypercalcemia.—This shortens the ST segment without affecting the duration of the T wave, with resulting shortening of QTc (see Fig 6–11).

    3. Hypokalemia.—This produces one of the least specific ECG changes. When serum K is below 2.5 mEq/L, ECG changes consist of the following (Fig 6–12):

        a. Prominent U wave. There is an apparent prolongation of QTc, but actually a "long" QU interval is present.
        b. Flat or diphasic T waves.
        c. ST segment depression.

    With further lowering of serum K, the PR interval may become prolonged and sinoatrial block may occur.

    All of the ECG features of hypokalemia may be found in LVH with "strain," including prominent U waves. In LVH with "strain" the ST segment shift is usually toward the right and anteriorly, whereas in hypokalemia the ST segment shift is toward the left and posteriorly. Both hypokalemia and digitalis produce ST segment depression. Digitalis, however, produces a short QT interval and ordinarily no prominence of the U wave.

4. Hyperkalemia.—A tall, peaked, symmetric T wave with a narrow base, the so called "tented" T wave is the earliest ECG abnormality. In hyperkalemia, sinoatrial (SA) block, second-degree AV block (either Mobitz I or II), and passive or accelerated junctional or ventricular escape rhythm may be present. Severe hyperkalemia may result in either ventricular fibrillation or arrest. The following ECG sequence is associated with a progressive increase in the serum K level (see Fig 6–12). These changes are usually best seen in leads II, III, and left precordial leads.

    a. Tall "tented" T wave, usually best seen in precordial leads.

    b. Prolongation of QRS duration (intraventricular block).

    c. Prolongation of PR interval.

    d. Disappearance of P wave.

    e. Wide, bizarre, diphasic QRS complex ("sine wave").

    f. Ventricular fibrillation or cardiac arrest.

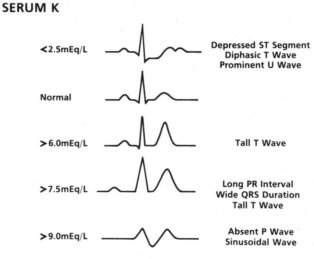

FIG 6–12.
ECG findings of hypokalemia and hyperkalemia.

REVIEW QUESTIONS

1. Which type of electrolyte imbalance is most likely present in the ECG tracing (lead II) from a newborn male infant shown in Figure 6–13?

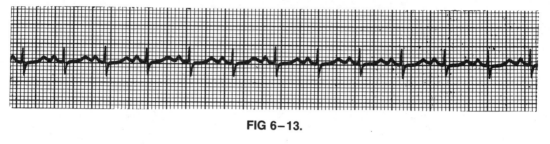

FIG 6–13.

   a. Hypocalcemia
   b. Hypercalcemia
   c. Hypokalemia
   d. Hyperkalemia
   e. Hypocalcemia and hyperkalemia

2. Which of the following shortens the QT interval (QTc)?
   a. Digitalis
   b. Hypocalcemia
   c. Left ventricular hypertrophy
   d. Hypokalemia

3. Which of the following statements is correct regarding myocardial infarction?
   a. The initial QRS vector moves away from the area of infarction.
   b. The T vector moves toward the infarction.
   c. Low QRS voltages throughout the limb leads are frequent findings.
   d. The pathologic Q waves are present only during the acute phase.

Answer the following questions either "true" or "false."

4. Prolongation of PR intervals (first-degree AV block) is always an indication of myocarditis.   True   False
5. Pericarditis is often associated with low-voltage QRS complexes in the limb leads.   True   False
6. Hypercalcemia is characterized by an ECG finding of tall, peaked T waves.   True   False
7. Hypocalcemia produces a prolongation of the QT interval, more specifically of the ST segment.   True   False
8. Prominent U waves are often seen in hypokalemia.   True   False
9. ST segment shifts of up to 2 mm in the precordial leads may be normal as long as they are of a junctional type (J-depression).   True   False
10. Shortening of the QTc interval is the earliest ECG sign of digitalis effect.   True   False
11. In anterolateral myocardial infarction the pathologic Q waves will be seen on leads III and aVF.   True   False
12. Elevated ST segment may be seen in pericarditis and myocardial infarction.   True   False

Answers may be found on page 239.

CHAPTER 7

Arrhythmias

The frequency and clinical significance of arrhythmias (other than sinus) differ in children and adults. Arrhythmias are relatively infrequent in infants and children. Because more adults have coronary arteriosclerotic heart disease, ventricular arrhythmias, for example, are more common, more serious, and of more complex mechanism than are those in children. However, increasing number of infants and children who survive surgical procedures for congenital heart defects develop arrhythmias, some complex, requiring treatment. In this chapter, only the basic arrhythmias with clearly defined mechanisms are presented with a brief discussion of clinical significance and treatment when applicable. Actual tracings of arrhythmias and AV conduction disturbances for readers to practice, along with author's interpretations, are presented in Chapter 10.

In normal sinus rhythm the sinoatrial (SA) node impulse depolarizes the right and left atria. The impulse then passes through the atrioventricular (AV) node at a much slower velocity than through any other portion of the heart (Table 7–1). Once it reaches the bundle of His, the conduction velocity becomes very fast and the impulse spreads simultaneously down the right and left bundle branches and the Purkinje fibers to depolarize the ventricular myocardium (see Chaps. 1 and 5 and the discussion later in this chapter). There are two other levels of potential pacemaker sites: the AV node (NH region) and the ventricle (Purkinje fibers). These lower pacemaker sites have a progressively slower rate of automaticity than that of the SA node and therefore do not compete with the SA node when all three pacemakers function normally. However, in the event of SA node failure or excessive slowing, a lower pacemaker site takes over the pacemaker function (escape beat). Occasionally, abnormal acceleration of the lower pacemakers will allow them to capture the pacemaker role.

TABLE 7–1.

Conduction Velocity

Atrial myocardium	1000 mm/sec
AV node	200 mm/sec
His-Purkinje system	4000 mm/sec
Ventricular myocardium	400 mm/sec

MECHANISMS OF ABNORMAL P WAVE AND QRS COMPLEX

Before discussing each arrhythmia, let us consider some basic principles that will aid in understanding the mechanisms of abnormal P waves and QRS complexes in various arrhythmias.

Importance of P Vector

The P wave represents atrial depolarization. The P axis (or vector) tells us the direction of atrial depolarization, and helps us identify the site of the pacemaker. Figure 7–1 illustrates with four examples how different P axes are used in deducing the pacemaker site.

1. In *sinus rhythm* the atrial depolarization wave spreads from the sinus node located in the right upper part of the atria in a leftward and downward direction. This produces a P axis +40 to +60 degrees (with a range of 0 to +90 degrees) with upright P waves in leads II and aVF and negative P waves in lead aVR (Fig 7–1,A).

2. If there is an abnormal pacemaker in the lower part of the atria, the wave of atrial depolarization will spread superiorly (Fig 7–1,B). This will produce an abnormal, *superiorly directed P axis* with negative P waves in leads II and aVF ("coronary sinus" rhythm).

3. If the location of the pacemaker changes from one point to another in the atria, the direction of the atrial depolarization (P axis) will change and so will the PR interval. This will produce a change in the shape of the P waves and PR interval *(wandering atrial pacemaker)* (Fig 7–1,C).

4. A P axis in the right lower quadrant is characteristic of patients with dextrocardia and situs inversus totalis (mirror-image dextrocardia) in which the right-to-left relationship is reversed (Fig 7–1,D).

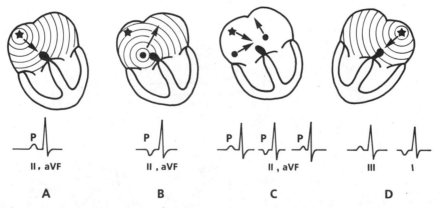

FIG 7–1.
Direction of atrial depolarization in normal and abnormal conditions. QRS complexes below each drawing are those anticipated to be present in particular leads. **A,** normal; **B,** low atrial ("coronary sinus") rhythm; **C,** wandering atrial pacemaker; **D,** mirror-image dextrocardia.

AV Node as an Impulse Generator

The AV node is considered to consist of three portions (Fig 7–2):

1. The upper atrionodal region *(AN region).*
2. The middle nodal region *(N region).*
3. The lower node-His region *(NH region).*

Intracellular recordings suggest that the upper and middle regions do not function as a pacemaker. The NH region is the only part of the node with demonstrated ability to pace the heart.

If the lower part of the AV node or upper His bundle (NH region) initiates the impulse, the normal antegrade QRS complex will be recorded. The superiorly directed P wave will follow slightly after the onset of the QRS complex because of the conduction delay provided by the AN and N regions (the delay in conduction is present in both antegrade and retrograde conduction through the AN and N regions). However, if the QRS and P waves occur simultaneously, the P waves will be obscured.

Since the upper and middle parts of the AV node do not demonstrate slow depolarization in diastole, the main characteristic of pacemaker tissue, many cardiologists have abandoned the term *nodal rhythm* in favor of the noncommittal term AV *junctional rhythm.* Since the NH and upper His bundle have been shown to be able to pace, it seems better either to retain the term nodal or to use *NH rhythm* or *His rhythm.*

Ventricle as an Impulse Generator

If the impulse reaches both ventricles through the normal His-Purkinje system, the time required to depolarize the entire ventricle is short (0.08 second in the adult and even shorter in the child) and a normal, narrow QRS complex results. If, however, an abnormal focus in either ventricle initiates depolarization, it takes much longer to depolarize both ventricles, since the conduction velocity through the ventricular myocardium is ten times slower than that through the His-Purkinje system (see Table 7–1). Therefore, the QRS duration becomes prolonged. If the ectopic focus is in the RV, the QRS complex resembles that of left bundle branch block (LBBB) since the LV is the last to be depolarized. An ectopic focus in the LV will produce an RBBB type of QRS complex for the same reason. The P wave does not precede the QRS complex and may or may not follow it.

FIG 7–2.
Diagram of the AV node and bundle of His. Conduction delay in the AV node is provided by the AN and N regions. Only the NH region has pacemaker capability.

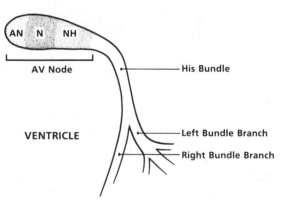

BASIC ARRHYTHMIAS

Only the common arrhythmias are discussed in this section, according to the origin of the impulse. A further exercise session is provided in Chapter 10.

Rhythms Originating in the Sinus Node

All rhythms that originate in the sinoatrial node (*sinus rhythm,* the normal rhythm at any age) have the following characteristics:

1. P waves preceding each QRS complex, with a regular PR interval. (The PR interval may be prolonged in first-degree AV block, as discussed later, but it is still a sinus mechanism.)
2. Normal P axis (0 to +90 degrees). This produces an upright P in lead II and an inverted P in aVR (see Fig 7–1,A).

Regular Sinus Rhythm
The rhythm is regular and the rate is normal for the patient's age. The characteristics of sinus rhythm are present (Fig 7–3).

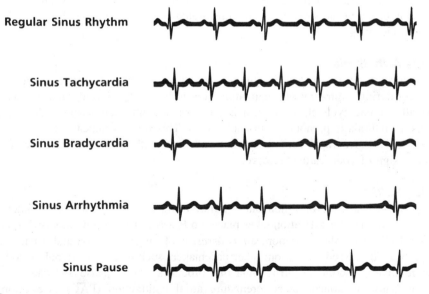

FIG 7–3.
Normal and abnormal rhythms originating in the SA node. All these rhythms have a P wave in front of each QRS complex with a regular PR interval and a P axis in the 0 to +90 degree quadrant.

Sinus Tachycardia

The rate is faster than normal for the patient's age, and the P-QRS complexes are perfectly normal. In adults, a rate in excess of 100 beats per minute is considered tachycardia. In general, a rate in excess of 140 per minute in children and a rate of 160 or more in infants may be significant.

In children, sinus tachycardia is usually due to anxiety created by undergoing an ECG and therefore is not as significant as it is in adults, unless it occurs during sleep. Tachycardia during sleep or at rest can be caused by congestive heart failure secondary to congenital or acquired heart disease, myocardial disease, fever, thyrotoxicosis, or shock. Treatment is required not for the tachycardia but for the underlying disorder.

Sinus Bradycardia

The rate is slower than normal for the patient's age, and the ECG complexes are completely normal. In adults, a rate under 60 beats per minute is defined as bradycardia. The definition is not clear-cut for pediatric patients, but a rate under 80 per minute in newborn infants and under 70 per minute in older children may be significant. During sinus bradycardia the AV node may capture the pacing role by virtue of a higher rate of automaticity.

Sinus bradycardia is rare in healthy children but is seen in trained athletes. Increased intracranial pressure, hypothyroidism, hypothermia, profound hypoxia, "sick sinus" syndrome, hyperkalemia, and drugs such as digitalis and beta-adrenergic blockers may cause sinus bradycardia. Sinus bradycardia per se rarely requires treatment, but treatment should be directed to correct an underlying cause.

Sinus Arrhythmia

Sinus arrhythmia is a phasic irregularity of the heart rate, increasing during inspiration and slowing during expiration but maintaining the normal P-QRS configuration and relation. Occasionally minute cycle changes occur in the P wave configuration and in the PR interval.

Sinus arrhythmia is pronounced in adolescents. This rhythm indicates that the cardiovascular system is under vagal control and not under sympathetic control and therefore is regarded as a sign of good cardiac reserve.

Sinus Pause

Sinus pause is a result of a momentary failure of the SA node to initiate an impulse. Neither atrial nor ventricular activation takes place; no P wave or QRS complex is recorded. It is, however, of relatively short duration. *Sinus arrest* is of longer duration and usually results in an escape beat (discussed later) from other pacemakers such as the junctional or nodal tissue. Another relatively uncommon arrhythmia that produces a long pause and causes confusion with sinus pause is nonconducted premature atrial contraction (PAC) (see ectopic atrial rhythm).

These sinus pauses may be due to increased vagal tone, hypoxia, or digitalis. They rarely need treatment except in the sick sinus syndrome (discussed below).

Sick Sinus Syndrome

Sick sinus syndrome (SSS), a well-known entity in adults, is now increasingly recognized in children who undergo extensive cardiac surgery, particularly that involving the atria and atrial septum such as the Mustard or Senning procedure for transposition of the great arteries. Rarely, the syndrome occurs secondary to arteritis or focal myocarditis or may be familial.

The sinus node may fail to function as the dominant pacemaker of the heart, or at least perform abnormally slowly, resulting in a variety of arrhythmias, with or without symptoms. The arrhythmias include profound sinus bradycardia, sinoatrial exit block, sinus arrest with junctional escape, paroxysmal atrial tachycardia, slow or fast ectopic atrial or nodal rhythm, and bradytachyarrhythmia. The rhythm may vary from one type to another; the abrupt slowing after tachycardia is the most worrisome, since overdrive suppression of the AV node can last long enough for syncope to occur. There is an increased frequency of AV nodal disorders in a population with SSS, which makes this a more ominous likelihood.

Patients who suffer from SSS in the immediate postoperative period may have frequent episodes of tachycardia, requiring antiarrhythmic drugs such as propranolol. Frequency of tachycardia tends to decrease over the years. Children with periods of extreme bradycardia following tachycardia may require demand pacemaker therapy. However, there is no current technology that will accelerate the atrial rate beyond a programmed but fixed rate, in contrast to the situation with normal sinus rhythm and complete AV block, with atrial sensing.

Rhythms Originating in the Atrium (Other Than SA Node), Ectopic Atrial Rhythm

The term *ectopy* or *ectopic beat* is used to signify the nonsinus rhythm in which other parts of the heart, rather than the SA node, are the pacemakers. Ectopic beats are usually premature but may come after a longer than normal pause (escape beat). Ectopic beats may be atrial, AV junctional, or ventricular in origin.

Atrial arrhythmias are characterized by the following:

1. P waves of unusual contour and/or an abnormal number per QRS complex,
2. QRS complexes of normal duration but with occasional bizarre, wide QRS complexes due to aberrancy (further discussion follows).

Premature Atrial Contraction (PAC)

The beat comes prematurely, occurring before the next normal beat is due. The P wave morphology depends on the site of the atrial ectopic focus. When it is high in the atrium, the P axis is usually normal (upright P in II) and the PR interval is usually normal. Since the sinus node is depolarized by the atrial activation, the sinus node "clock" resets so that the RR interval following the premature QRS complex is usually normal with resulting incomplete compensatory pause; that is, the length of two cycles, including one premature beat, is less than the length of two normal cycles (Fig 7–4).

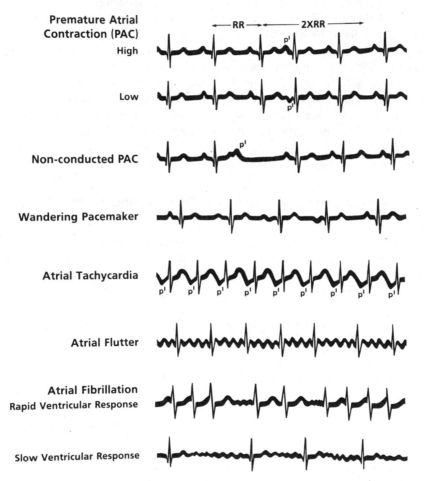

FIG 7–4.
Arrhythmias originating in the atrium.

When the ectopic focus is low in the atrium *(coronary sinus pacemaker),* the P axis is superiorly directed with upright P in aVR and negative P in II and aVF. The PR interval may be shorter than normal. There is an incomplete compensatory pause, as in the high atrial pacemaker (see Fig 7–4).

Occasionally the P wave will be buried in the T wave of the preceding beat, making it difficult to be certain whether the ectopy is of atrial or nodal origin. Rarely, a premature atrial contraction is not conducted to the ventricle, producing a long pause between two R waves. This requires a differentiation from sinus pause (see Fig 7–4). If the morphology of the premature P wave (P') is similar to the normal P wave, it resembles second-degree AV block. In non-conducted PAC, the PP' interval is shorter than the normal PP interval, whereas in second-degree AV block, the PP interval is unaltered.

Premature atrial contractions are common in healthy children, even in newborn infants, and may have no significance. They may also be associated with structural heart disease. PAC per se does not require treatment.

Wandering Pacemaker

A wandering pacemaker represents a gradual shift of the site of impulse formation through several cycles, from the SA node to the ectopic atrial focus or to the nodal pacemaker (see Fig 7–1,C). There are gradual changes in the configuration of P waves and PR intervals. The QRS complex is normal (see Fig 7–4). This is a benign arrhythmia and requires no treatment.

Atrial Tachycardia

Very rapid tachycardia (usually 240 ± 40 beats per minute), with normal-appearing QRS complexes, was formerly thought to be produced by rapid firing of a single focus in the atrium. At very rapid rates, the P wave is buried in the T of the preceding beat so that atrial tachycardia is difficult to separate from the more rare nodal tachycardia. This led to use of the term *supraventricular tachycardia* (SVT) to include both of these arrhythmias. Actually, the great majority of occurrences of SVT are due to AV reentry or reciprocating tachycardia (see Fig 7–6) rather than rapid firing of a single focus (see following discussion). Nevertheless, there *are* uncommon cases of nonreciprocating atrial tachycardia that originate from a single repetitive focus. These are distinguished by the term *ectopic atrial tachycardia.*

These patients with ectopic or nonreciprocating atrial tachycardia show a very regular rhythm over a brief interval, but during the course of a day, the rates vary substantially, whereas reciprocating AV tachycardia occurs in paroxysms of SVT. The ectopic atrial tachycardia patients also may develop second-degree AV block (see Fig 7–8) with 2:1 or 3:1 block, which clearly distinguishes the repetitive mechanism from the reciprocating mechanism. The ectopic atrial tachycardia tends to be chronic, and may be associated with sick sinus syndrome (see above). Treatment of ectopic atrial tachycardia may be difficult, since cessation of firing of the focus may be followed by profound bradycardia, or even asystole. If bradycardia is not a problem, propranolol may be effective, otherwise a demand pacemaker may be required.

Atrial Flutter

Atrial activity is seen as flutter or F waves with a "sawtooth" configuration, best seen in leads V1, II, and III. The atrial rate is about 300 per minute (240 to 360 per minute). The AV node cannot respond that rapidly, fortunately, so there is a degree of AV block (2:1, 3:1, 4:1, etc.). The QRS configuration is usually normal (see Fig 7–4).

Atrial flutter is rare in infants and children. It may be associated with structural heart disease with dilated atria, myocarditis, or other acute infectious disease. It may occur following intra-atrial surgery. Treatment consists of digoxin (to increase the AV block and slow the ventricular rate) with or without propranolol. Electrical cardioversion may be required. Quinidine may prevent recurrences.

Atrial Fibrillation

The atrial waves are totally irregular and vary in size and shape from beat to beat. They are usually most prominent in V1. The atrial rate ranges from 350 to 600 per minute. The ventricular response is irregularly irregular and may be fast or slow (see Fig 7–4). The QRS complexes are usually normal. A circus movement, entirely in the atrium, is the mechanism for most instances of fibrillation (as well as for atrial flutter).

Atrial fibrillation, like flutter, is rare in children. When present it is usually associated with structural heart defect or occurs following an intra-atrial surgical procedure. Treatment with digoxin is used initially to decrease ventricular rate. Propranolol may be added if necessary. Conversion to sinus rhythm is worth trying in an acute situation, either by countershock, with quinidine, or both.

Rhythms Originating in the AV Node

Rhythms originating in the AV nodal or junctional area are characterized by the following:

1. The P waves may be absent, or if present they occur after the QRS complex and are inverted.
2. The QRS complex is usually normal in duration and configuration.

Nodal Premature Beat

A normal QRS complex occurs prematurely with or without inverted (retrogradely conducted) P′ wave following the QRS complex. There may or may not be a complete compensatory pause, depending on whether the SA node is discharged prematurely by a retrograde activation of the atria. If the SA node is discharged, the compensatory pause is incomplete as a result of resetting the SA node "clock" (Fig 7–5). If the SA node is not discharged, the compensatory pause is complete.

Single, infrequent nodal premature beats have no clinical significance.

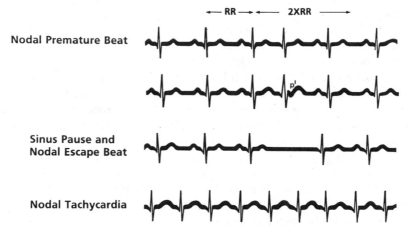

FIG 7–5.
Arrhythmias originating in the AV node.

Nodal Escape Beat

Among potential pacemaker sites (the sinus node, the AV node, and the ventricles) the AV node (or NH region) has the second fastest pacemaker rate, with the SA node having the fastest rate. If the SA node impulse fails to reach the AV node in time, the AV node will spontaneously depolarize. This is called a nodal (junctional) escape beat (see Fig 7–5). The escape beat will come later than the anticipated normal beat, and there will be a normal QRS complex with or without an inverted P wave following it. If there is a persistent failure or slowing of the SA node, a slow *AV junctional rhythm* may continue at a rate of 40 to 60.

Transient or sustained junctional rhythms are common after a surgical procedure involving the atria, particularly after the Mustard or Senning procedure for the transposition of the great arteries. These rhythms generally require no specific treatment, although the rates occasionally are slow enough to require a demand pacemaker.

Accelerated Nodal Rhythm

If the sinus rate and AV conduction are normal, and the AV node (NH region) with enhanced automaticity has captured the pacemaking role at a faster rate (60 to 120), the rhythm is described as accelerated nodal (or AV junctional) rhythm. Treatment is not usually necessary, but if the patient is receiving digoxin, digitalis toxicity is likely and the dose should be reduced.

Nodal Tachycardia

The rate can vary from 120 to 200 per minute. The QRS complex is usually normal and regular, although aberrant conduction may develop, as in atrial tachycardia (further discussion on aberrancy follows). The inverted P' wave may or may not follow QRS complex (see Fig 7–5). It may be difficult to separate nodal from atrial tachycardia. Therefore, the atrial, nodal, and reciprocating AV tachycardias are grouped as *supraventricular tachycardia* (SVT).

Treatment may not be necessary if the rate is less than 130. Although digoxin is the drug of choice for most cases of supraventricular tachycardia, it is contraindicated in a true form of nodal tachycardia. In that instance, quinidine is probably the drug of choice.

Aberrancy

When a supraventricular impulse prematurely reaches the AV node or bundle of His, it may find one bundle branch excitable and the other still refractory. It will be conducted down only one bundle branch, resulting in a QRS pattern of BBB. The right bundle branch usually has a longer refractory period than the left bundle branch, producing QRS complexes similar to those of RBBB. This phenomenon is therefore dependent on an unequal refractory period of the bundle branches and premature impulse formation. In addition, a long preceding RR interval paradoxically predisposes aberrancy; a long RR interval makes the subsequent refractory period relatively long (Ashman phenomenon).

Supraventricular rhythm with aberrant ventricular conduction is difficult to differentiate from arrhythmias of ventricular origin with wide QRS complexes. Fortunately, aberrancy is uncommon in children. Therefore, wide QRS tachycardia without visible P waves should be considered ventricular tachycardia until proved otherwise. The features suggesting an aberrancy are based on both the QRS morphology and the relationship of the P wave and QRS complex.

QRS Morphology.— There is usually an rsR' pattern in V1 and qRs pattern in V6, since most examples of aberrant conduction resemble RBBB. Furthermore, the QRS complex of ventricular origin is completely bizarre and does not resemble the classic forms of either RBBB or LBBB.

P-QRS Relationship.— The bizarre QRS complexes must be shown to be related to preceding P waves in order to make a diagnosis of aberrancy. If the QRS complexes are dissociated from the P waves, an ectopic ventricular rhythm is probably present. If the QRS complexes are related to the P waves, it may be either an aberration or a ventricular ectopy with retrograde AV conduction in which the P wave follows rather than precedes the QRS complex. In this situation the inspection of a rhythm strip showing the beginning of the arrhythmia may be diagnostic; the presence of a P wave in front of the very first aberrant QRS complex favors aberrancy.

AV Reentrant Tachycardia

Reciprocating (reentry) AV tachycardia (RAVT) is the most common mechanism of supraventricular tachycardia. In ectopic atrial tachycardia, increased automacity of an ectopic pacemaker is the mechanism. In supraventricular tachycardia (SVT) due to reentry, two pathways are involved, at least one of which is the AV node, connecting the atria and ventricles in a continuous, circus-type circuit. The other, accessory pathway, may be anatomically separate, such as the bundle of Kent (see Fig 5–15), or only functionally separate, as in a dual AV node pathway. Patients with accessory pathways frequently, but not inevitably, have preexcitation (see Chap. 5).

Accessory Reciprocating AV Tachycardia

The earliest understood example of reciprocating AV tachycardia is the SVT that occurs in the Wolff-Parkinson-White syndrome. When the conduction velocity is faster in the accessory fibers than in the AV node, as is usual for the bundle of Kent, the ventricle that receives the termination of the fibers will be preexcited. However, the recovery time for the Kent bundle is widely variable, sometimes longer than for the AV node. If an atrial extrasystole occurs, the prematurity of the extrasystole may find the accessory bundle refractory, but the AV node may conduct, producing a normal QRS; when the impulse reaches the Kent bundle from

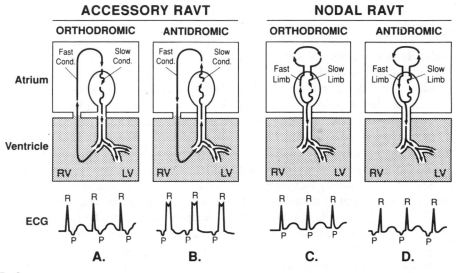

ACCESSORY RAVT

ORTHODROMIC   ANTIDROMIC

NODAL RAVT

ORTHODROMIC   ANTIDROMIC

A.   B.   C.   D.

FIG 7–6.

Diagram showing the mechanisms of reciprocating AV tachycardia *(RAVT)* in relation to ECG findings. In orthodromic RAVT **(A)**, the ventricles are excited normally through the normal *(slow)* path of the AV node. The atria are excited through the accessory bundle, producing retrograde (inverted) P waves following QRS complexes with a long PR interval (and a short RP interval). The QRS complex is narrow. This is the most common mechanism of SVT in patients with WPW syndrome. In antidromic accessory RAVT **(B)**, wide QRS complexes with LBBB pattern develop if the accessory bundle terminates in the RV. Retrograde P waves precede the QRS complex with a short PR interval (and a long RP interval).

In the orthodromic nodal RAVT (common form) **(C)**, retrograde P waves are usually concealed in the QRS complex, although they may appear following it with a very short RP interval. The QRS duration is narrow, following orthodromic conduction in the normal *(slow)* path of the AV node. In the antidromic nodal RAVT (uncommon) **(D)**, narrow QRS complexes will be preceded by retrograde P waves, excited antidromically through the normal AV pathway, with a short PR and a long RP interval. Note that the ECG in this situation is similar to that of ectopic atrial tachycardia. See text for further discussion. *LV:* left ventricle; *RV:* right ventricle.

the ventricular side, the bundle will have recovered, and allow reentry into the atrium. The retrograde activation of the atrium will be demonstrated by a P vector that is superiorly directed, although the P wave may be difficult to detect because it follows closely the QRS. In turn, the cycle is maintained by reentry into the AV node, with a very short RR interval. The resulting SVT is paroxysmal, with an abrupt onset and termination, unlike the ectopic atrial tachycardia, which is more chronic and variable in rate. Note that there is a short RP interval for the RAVT in contrast to the short PR for atrial tachycardia. When the QRS is normal, common in WPW during tachycardia, the rhythm is called *orthodromic reciprocating AV tachycardia* (Fig 7–6,A). Less common is a widened QRS complex, which usually indicates that the conduction into the ventricle (antegrade) is via the accessory bundle, and the reentry into the atrium is retrograde via the AV node (Fig 7–5,B). In this case, the tachyrhythmia is called *antidromic reciprocating AV tachycardia*. It should be obvious from considering these diagrams that a premature ventricular contraction (PVC) could initiate antidromic RAVT, but the actual outcome would depend upon the prematurity of the PVC as well as the recovery times of the two limbs of the potential reentry cycle.

Other types of accessory fibers (James, Mahaim) were shown in Figure 5–15. There is increasing doubt that they are causally related to RAVT; they are probably "innocent bystanders" in most cases. However, these tracts may be of significance in relation to the rare (in pediatric experience) event of atrial fibrillation when they may transmit rapidly to the ventricles, without block, if their recovery times are short.

Nodal Reciprocating AV Tachycardia

Dual or discontinuous pathways in the AV node are more common than accessory bundles, at least as functional entities. For these dual nodal tracts to be of clinical importance, their involvement in symptomatic tachyrhythmia must be demonstrated, since their presence can be demonstrated in approximately 40% of asymptomatic children by electrophysiologic studies, and in 10% to 20% of normal adults. On the other hand, 80% of children with nodal reentry AV tachycardia demonstrate dual AV node pathways. For SVT to occur, the two pathways would have to have, at least temporarily, different conduction and recovery rates, creating the substrate for a reentry tachycardia. Fig 7–6,C illustrates the common form of nodal reciprocating AV tachycardia with dual pathways in the AV node, in which the normal, slow pathway through the AV node is utilized in antegrade conduction to the His bundles (orthodromic), creating a normal appearing QRS. Note that the P vector would be the same as for SVT associated with WPW, although the RP interval will be very short, causing it to be superimposed on the QRS, or with a very short RP interval. Consequently, the differential diagnosis between nodal and accessory types of orthodromic RAVT would have to await conversion from the SVT; after conversion the patient with the accessory type of RAVT would have the characteristic features diagrammed in Figure 5–15.

In the uncommon form of nodal RAVT, the fast tract of the AV node transmits the antegrade impulse to the bundle of His, and the normal, slow pathway of the AV node transmits antidromically. The resulting SVT demonstrates a short PR, an inverted P, and a normal QRS (Fig 7–6,D). Thus, the two forms of nodal RAVT will both demonstrate a normal QRS; in the antidromic form the QRS will be preceded by an inverted P, whereas in the common dual nodal RAVT (orthodromic) the QRS will be followed shortly by the inverted P, if it is not obscured by the QRS. Note the similarity of the antidromic nodal RAVT to ectopic atrial tachycardia; clinically, the former is paroxysmal, and the latter is more chronic and with a more variable rate.

There are instances demonstrated by electrophysiologic studies (EPS) in which there appears to be enhanced or accelerated conduction in one of the two nodal pathways, which could result in an ECG that resembles the LGL syndrome, with a short PR during sinus rhythm but a wide-QRS with tachycardia.

In any of the reentrant tachycardias, it should be noted that any type of AV block is incompatible with RAVT. AV block would abruptly terminate the tachycardia, at least temporarily.

As mentioned above, bundle branch block patterns may develop with RAVT, which may produce wide-QRS tachycardia, increasing the difficulty of diagnosis. Also, the accessory pathways may demonstrate unidirectional block, which may mask the existence of the accessory fibers. It is clear, however, that the presence of paroxysmal SVT always indicates the presence of some second connection between the atria and ventricles. There are also occasional patients with multiple accessory AV connections.

RAVT is usually responsive to treatment, and if the paroxysm lasts more than an hour or two, treatment is increasingly urgent. When it is long-lasting (more than 24 hours), congestive heart failure may supervene and the clinical picture may mimic pneumonia or sepsis. It may be seen both in normal children (about 50% of cases) and in those with congenital heart disease. Nonspecific febrile illness may precipitate it. About 20% of children with SVT show ECG evidence of preexcitation when they do not have the tachycardia.

When the SVT has been of brief duration, maneuvers to increase vagal tone may succeed in converting the SVT to sinus rhythm. If these maneuvers fail, the treatment of choice is digitalization in the pediatric age group. In a critically ill infant with severe congestive heart failure, cardioversion may be used initially. Cardioversion may also be used initially in a patient with wide QRS complexes in which differentiation between ventricular tachycardia and supraventricular tachycardia with aberrancy is difficult. Maneuvers that increase vagal tone, such as carotid sinus massage or gagging, are seldom successful in sick infants with congestive heart failure but may be successful after digitalization. These maneuvers, the Valsalva maneuver, vigorous coughing, and wet stimulation of the face (dive reflex) may be effective in older children, particularly with tachycardia of short duration. Abrupt increase in blood pressure by intravenous infusion of methoxamine or phenylephrine often converts the arrhythymias by reflex increase in vagal tone. Intravenous administration of verapamil (a calcium channel blocker) or propranolol is certainly not the treatment of choice; these drugs often produce extreme bradycardia and hypotension in infants, requiring resuscitative measures. Adenosine is rapidly becoming popular, since its effect is quite brief, but highly successful. It is given as 0.05 mg/kg intravenously; a repeat dose is given in 1 minute, if necessary, increasing the dose up to 0.25 mg/kg.

After conversion to normal sinus rhythm has been accomplished, these children may be maintained on a regimen of digoxin for some months to prevent recurrent tachycardia. Although digoxin does not actually prevent the attack, it facilitates spontaneous conversion. In patients with WPW syndrome, propranolol, with or without digoxin, may be an effective agent in preventing further attacks. However, many children will have only brief episodes of tachycardia, and the episodes may be infrequent. Daily medications for these patients may be unnecessary. Many can be managed with ad hoc treatment (for conversion only, without maintenance), or no medications at all. In the rare case where medical management fails in patients with WPW syndrome, surgical interruption of accessory pathways should be considered.

Rhythms Originating in the Ventricle

Ventricular arrhythmias are characterized by the following:

1. QRS complexes are bizarre in configuration and long in duration.
2. QRS complexes and T waves often point in opposite directions.
3. QRS complexes are randomly related to P waves, and fusion beats are common.

Premature Ventricular Contraction (PVC)

A PVC is characterized by a bizarre, wide QRS complex occurring before the next expected QRS complex in a regular rhythm. The T wave points in the direction opposite to the QRS complex. There is no premature P wave preceding the premature QRS complex. The retrograde impulse is usually blocked in the atrioventricular node, and the SA node is not depolarized by the retrograde conduction; the SA node "clock" keeps its original pace. Therefore, there is a full compensatory pause. This means that the length of two cycles, including one premature beat, is the same length as two normal cycles ($2 \times RR$) (Fig 7–7). If the PVC arises from a single focus *(unifocal),* the QRS complexes will be of the same configuration in the same lead. If they arise from different foci *(multifocal),* the QRS complexes will be of different configurations in the same lead. If each PVC alternates with normal ventricular complexes regularly, the rhythm is called *ventricular bigeminy or coupling.* If each PVC regularly follows two normal QRS complexes, the rhythm is called *ventricular trigeminy.* (Some reserve the term for one normal QRS followed by two PVCs, the latter called *couplets.*)

Occasional PVCs are benign in children, particularly if they disappear or decrease in number with exercise. Multifocal and frequent PVCs, particularly couplets, those precipitated by activity, and those associated with an underlying cardiac condition are usually significant. Antiarrhythmic drugs such as lidocaine, quinidine, propranolol, diphenylhydantoin, or procainamide may be indicated.

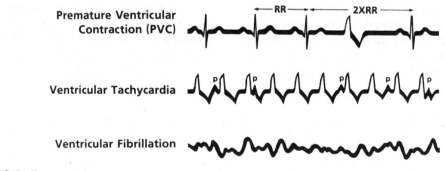

FIG 7–7.
Ventricular arrhythmias.

Ventricular Tachycardia (VT)

Ventricular tachycardia is a series of three or more premature ventricular contractions (PVCs) occurring at a rate of 120 to 180 per minute (see Fig 7–7). It is difficult to differentiate VT from supraventricular tachycardia with aberrant (intraventricular) conduction (see section on aberrancy for full discussion). A reliable sign of ventricular arrhythmia is the presence of a *ventricular fusion complex*. This is a QRS complex that is produced in part by a normally conducted supraventricular impulse and in part by an ectopic ventricular impulse. The resulting QRS complex is intermediate in appearance between the patient's normal conducted beat and the pure ectopic ventricular beat. Since aberrancy is rare in children, wide QRS tachycardia without visible P waves should be considered VT.

Ventricular tachycardia is rare in children but is a serious arrhythmia and may signify myocardial damage or dysfunction. It can deteriorate to a ventricular fibrillation, although this is not as likely as in the adult with coronary artery disease. Faster rates should be treated promptly with antiarrhythmic drugs such as IV lidocaine. Cardioversion is rarely of more than transient effectiveness. Complete abolition of the arrhythmia is less important than keeping the rate below 150 for infants, and 130 for older children.

Ventricular Fibrillation (VF)

Ventricular fibrillation is characterized by a bizarre ventricular QRS pattern of varying size and configuration. The rate is rapid and irregular (see Fig 7–7). This is usually a terminal arrhythmia as it cannot provide effective perfusion of the myocardium. Successful resuscitation depends on prompt recognition and cardiac defibrillation.

DISTURBANCES OF AV CONDUCTION

Atrioventricular block (AV block) is a disturbance in conduction between the normal sinus impulse and the eventual ventricular response. Depending on the severity of the conduction disturbance, AV block is classified into three classes: (1) A simple prolongation of the PR interval is called *first-degree AV block;* (2) *second-degree AV block* is an intermediate grade of conduction disturbance in which some atrial impulses are not conducted into the ventricle; (3) *third-degree AV block* (or complete heart block) is the most extreme form of AV block in which none of the atrial impulses are conducted into the ventricle (Fig 7–8).

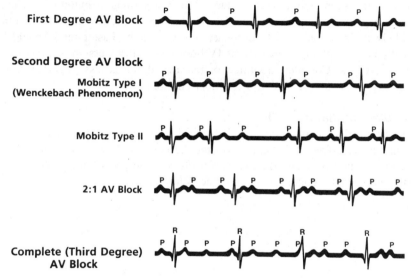

FIG 7–8.
Disturbances of atrioventricular conduction.

First-Degree AV Block

In first-degree AV block there is a disturbance in conduction between the sinus node and the ventricles, produced by an abnormal delay in conduction through the AV node. This results in prolongation of the PR interval beyond the upper limit of normal for the patient's age and rate (see Table 3–1). Sinus rhythm is maintained and no dropped beats occur. The QRS complex is normal in configuration (see Fig 7–8).

It is sometimes seen in healthy children and in children with infectious disease. It is sometimes associated with a wide variety of cardiac conditions such as rheumatic fever, cardiomyopathies, atrial septal defect, and Ebstein's anomaly. It is also a sign of digitalis toxicity. First-degree AV block (not caused by digitalis) does not produce symptoms or require treatment.

Second-Degree AV Block

Second-degree AV block is characterized by some, but not all, dropped beats in which some P waves are not followed by QRS complexes. There are several types:

Mobitz Type I (Wenckebach Block or Phenomenon).—There is a progressive lengthening of the PR interval culminating in a dropped ventricular beat (over three to six cycles); a long diastolic pause results and the cycle is then resumed. The number of beats in each cycle is not necessarily constant. The QRS complexes are normal in configuration (see Fig 7–8). Type I block with a normal QRS complex almost always takes place at the level of the AV node. It may be a sign of digitalis toxicity and can occur in any condition that causes first-degree AV block.

Mobitz Type II.—The AV conduction is "all or none." There is either normal AV conduction with normal PR interval, or the conduction is completely blocked. The atrial rate is normal, but the ventricular rate depends strictly on the number of successfully conducted atrial impulses. The failure is at the His bundle level.

This type of second-degree AV block is more serious than type I since it may progress to complete heart block. Prophylactic pacemaker therapy may be indicated in older adults who could not survive sudden, complete heart block.

Two-to-One (or Higher) AV Block.—A ventricular complex follows every second (third or fourth) atrial complex, resulting in 2:1 (3:1 or 4:1) AV block. The atrial rate (PP interval) and the PR interval of the conducted beat are normal (see Fig 7–8). These are usually due to Mobitz I mechanism (block in the AV node), particularly when associated with normal QRS complexes, but a His bundle recording may be necessary to determine whether the block occurs in the upper AV node or at the level of the His bundle, in occasional cases.

Complete (Third-Degree) AV Block

In complete AV block, the atria and ventricles beat entirely independently of one another. The atrial rhythm is regular (regular PP interval) and the rate is that of the average sinus rhythm for the patient's age. The ventricular rate is also quite regular (regular RR interval) but of much slower rate. The QRS complex is normal if the pacemaker is in the AV node or a level higher than the bifurcation of the His bundle (see Fig 7–8). Most children with congenital complete heart block belong in this category. The QRS complexes will have the appearance of ventricular premature beats if the pacemaker is in either ventricle with a slow rate (about 40/min), called *idioventricular rhythm*. Surgically induced or acquired (postmyocardial infarction) third-degree heart block may be of this type. Thus the QRS complex is commonly of normal duration in congenital complete heart block, whereas it is usually prolonged in surgically induced or acquired third-degree AV block.

Congenital complete heart block may be an isolated anomaly or may be associated with structural defects such as L-transposition of the great arteries. There is frequent association of maternal lupus erythematosus or mixed connective tissue disease with congenital complete heart block in the offspring. Asymptomatic childen with congenital heart block do not require pacemaker therapy until they become symptomatic. Surgically induced complete heart block may require pacemaker therapy, at least during the immediate postoperative period.

Atrioventricular Dissociation

Confusion has existed and still exists regarding the definition of atrioventricular (AV) dissociation. A widely accepted use of AV dissociation is any condition in which the atria and ventricles beat independently, so that the P waves and QRS complexes do not have any relationship. Such a dissociation may be caused by (1) slowed rate of the sinus node, which allows escape of a subsidiary or latent pacemaker; (2) accelerated rate of normally slower or latent pacemakers (AV node or ventricle); or (3) complete or advanced AV block. In this sense, AV dissociation is not a diagnosis and its cause should be clarified; for example, AV dissociation due to sinus bradycardia with nodal escape beats.

However, some authorities limit AV dissociation to the first two conditions excluding complete heart block, i.e., marked slowing of the sinus node or acceleration of the AV node. AV dissociation and complete AV block both demonstrate independence of the atria and ventricles, but the mechanisms underlying are so different that, at least, the mechanisms should be specified, since complete AV block has a more ominous prognosis.

In AV dissociation the atrial rate is slower than the ventricular rate, whereas in complete heart block the ventricular rate is usually slower than the atrial rate (Fig 7–9). In AV dissociation an atrial impulse may conduct to the AV node if it comes at the right time (see Fig 7–9). The conducted beats can be recognized by their relative prematurity. In complete AV block no atrial impulse goes through the AV node. Therefore, the RR interval maintains clock-like regularity, and the ventricular rate is relatively slow.

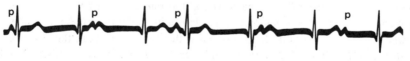

FIG 7–9.
AV dissociation owing to either marked slowing of the sinus node or acceleration of the AV node. The fourth complex is conducted, changing the rhythm (called "interference"). All of the other complexes originate in the AV node, where there is higher automaticity.

Digitalis Toxicity

Digitalization in children needs to be monitored closely by frequent rhythm strips, primarily to detect digitalis toxicity. The ECG does not answer the question of whether the patient is "fully" digitalized; it is a clinical decision. Findings suggestive of digitalis effect and those suggestive of toxicity are listed below. In general, digitalis effect is confined to ventricular repolarization, whereas toxicity involves disturbances in the formation and conduction of the impulse. Obviously, an ECG *before* starting digitalis therapy is mandatory.

Effect

1. Shortening of QTc, the earliest sign of digitalis effect.
2. Sagging ST segment and decreased T amplitude (see Fig 6–3,B).
3. Slowing of the heart rate.

Toxicity

1. Prolongation of PR interval is a more reliable early sign of toxicity than arrhythmias. It may progress to second-degree AV block. (Some normal children may have a prolonged PR interval.)
2. Profound sinus bradycardia or SA block.
3. Supraventricular arrhythmias, such as atrial or nodal ectopic beats, and tachycardia, particularly if accompanied by AV block, are more common than ventricular arrhythmias in children.
4. Ventricular bigeminy or trigeminy is extremely rare in children with digitalis toxicity, although common in adults. Premature ventricular contractions are not uncommon in children, however, and death may follow ventricular tachycardia.

A sound rule is to assume that any arrhythmia occurring *with* digitalis is *caused by* digitalis until proved otherwise.

REVIEW QUESTIONS

Answer the following questions either "true" or "false."

1. Shortening of the QTc interval is the earliest sign of digitalis toxicity.   True   False
2. The NH region is the only part of the AV node with demonstrated ability to pace the heart.   True   False
3. There is a full compensatory pause after a premature ventricular contraction (PVC).   True   False
4. The QRS complex is commonly of normal duration in congenital complete heart block whereas the QRS duration is usually prolonged in surgically induced heart block.   True   False
5. The Wolff-Parkinson-White syndrome is a frequent cause of sick sinus syndrome.   True   False
6. Treatment of choice for paroxysmal atrial tachycardia (PAT) is digitalization.   True   False
7. The conduction delay in the AV node is provided by the AV and N regions.   True   False
8. Prolongation of the PR interval is a more reliable early sign of digitalis toxicity than arrhythmias.   True   False
9. A wandering pacemaker is characterized by a gradual change in the shape and duration of the P waves as well as in the QRS complexes.   True   False
10. In sinus rhythm the P wave is upright in II and inverted in aVR.   True   False

11. Mobitz type II second-degree AV block is more serious than Mobitz type I (Wenckebach phenomenon) and may require prophylactic pacemaker therapy.   True   False

12. In complete heart block (third-degree AV block) the RR interval is of clock-like regularity and the ventricular rate is slower than the atrial rate.   True   False

Answers may be found on page 239.

CHAPTER 8

Chamber Localization

Although we generally assume that the cardiac chambers are positioned in normal anatomical relation to one another, there are occasional cases in which this assumption is wrong and the anatomical left ventricle is on the right side of the right ventricle or the anatomical right atrium is on the left side of the left atrium. An electrocardiogram may provide clues to these types of abnormalities. In this chapter we will consider some typical abnormalities of the right-to-left relationship of the cardiac chambers.

The heart and the great arteries can be viewed as three separate segments, i.e., the atria, the ventricles, and the great arteries (pulmonary artery and aorta). These three segments can vary from normal position either independently or together. Their exact relationship to one another can be confirmed only by echocardiography, angiocardiography, or morphological examination. Electrocardiography, however, can be helpful in predicting the location of the atria and the ventricles, though not the great arteries except by inference. Although the methods of locating the atria and ventricles by using ECGs are valid, there are many exceptions, with both false-positive results and false-negative results possible, particularly in locating the ventricles.

LOCATING THE ATRIA AND VENTRICLES

Locating the Atria

The sinoatrial (SA) node, marked by a star in Figure 8–1, is almost always located in the (anatomical) right atrium (RA). The P vector is directed to the opposite side of the SA node and inferiorly. Therefore, the atria can be located by the P axis of the electrocardiogram. For example, if the SA node (and therefore the RA) is in the right side, the P axis will be in the left lower quadrant (0 to +90 degrees), and if the SA node or the anatomical RA is located in the left side, as in mirror-image dextrocardia, the P axis will be in the right lower quadrant (+90 to +180 degrees) (see Fig 8–1).

Another way to locate the atria is to use x-ray films of the chest and upper abdomen. The RA and the liver are almost always on the same side. By echocardiography or angiocardiography, the inferior vena cava almost always identifies the right atrium, when the connection is identifiable.

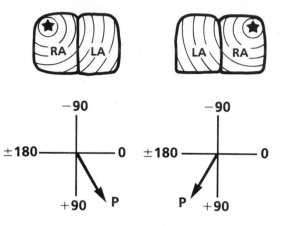

FIG 8–1.
Locating the atria by using the P axis. When the RA is on the right side, the P axis is in the left lower quadrant (0 to +90 degrees). When the RA is on the left side, the P axis is in the right lower quadrant (+90 to +180 degrees). This is based on the fact that the SA node is almost always located in the RA.

Locating the Ventricles

Provided there is a ventricular septum, the direction of its depolarization (see arrow in Fig 8–2) is from the embryonic left to the right ventricle. The Q waves represent the septal depolarization. In the normal situation in which the left ventricle is to the left of the right ventricle, the direction of the septal depolarization will be to the right, producing the Q waves in leads I, V5, and V6 (because the septal depolarization vector is moving away from the positive electrode of these leads). If the "left" ventricle is to the right of the right ventricle, the direction of the septal depolarization will be to the left. Therefore, the Q waves will be absent in leads I, V5, or V6. Instead, the Q waves will be present in the right-sided precordial leads, such as V1, V4R, or V6R, because the septal depolarization is moving away from the RPLs (see Fig 8–2). V4R and V6R are right-sided precordial leads that are obtained with chest electrodes positioned on the mirror-image points of V4 and V6.

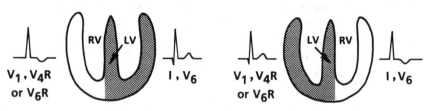

FIG 8–2.
Locating the ventricles. The left ventricle (LV) is usually located on the same side as the precordial leads that show Q waves. If V6 (left-sided) shows a Q wave, the LV is on the left side. If V4R or V6R shows a Q wave, the LV is to the right of the anatomical right ventricle.

LOCATING ABNORMAL CHAMBERS

The principles discussed above are helpful in identifying different types of dextrocardia (the situation in which the heart is predominantly right-sided), mesocardia (midline heart), and levocardia with abnormal chamber position such as L-transposition of the great arteries and single ventricle. Detailed discussion of the subject is beyond the scope of this book, but a brief, simplified discussion will be presented.

Heart in the Right Side of the Chest

When the heart is found to be in the right side of the chest on a chest roentgenogram, a cardiology consultation is usually obtained in order to clarify whether there is a structural abnormality or whether there is a simple mirror-image dextrocardia in association with situs inversus totalis. The abnormal position of the heart in the right side of the chest may be suspected on a routine ECG by the presence of progressive decrease in QRS amplitudes toward V6 (see Fig 8–4). X-ray films of the chest help in locating the atria, as previously discussed, in that they reveal the location of the liver. In general, the heart in the right side of the chest may be due to one of the following situations (Fig 8–3):

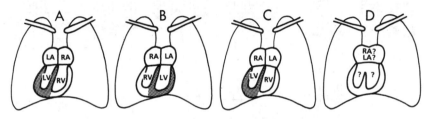

FIG 8–3.
Examples of common conditions when the apex of the heart is in the right chest.

1. Complete reversal of the right-to-left relationship, as in *mirror-image dextrocardia*. This is often seen in otherwise normal people with situs inversus totalis (Fig 8–3,A). The anterior-posterior relationships of the two ventricles are normal; only the right-to-left relationships are reversed.

The P axis is +90 to +180 degrees (right lower quadrant). Q waves are present in V5R and V6R, the right-sided chest leads. Figure 8–4 is an example of this type. Usually no structural anomaly is present. Dextrocardia of this type may be seen in Kartagener's syndrome (triad of situs inversus totalis, paranasal sinusitis, and bronchiectasis).

2. The apex of the heart is rotated toward the right side of the chest with the normal right-to-left relationship maintained, creating *dextroversion* (Fig 8–3,B). This displacement may be due to an extrinsic abnormality such as hypoplasia of the right lung.

The P axis remains in the normal quadrant (0 to +90 degrees) and Q waves are present in leads I, V5, and V6. The left-sided precordial leads (LPLs) show a progressive decrease in the QRS amplitude as they go farther from the heart. Right-sided chest leads, V5R and V6R, do not show Q waves. Figure 8–5 is an example of this type.

3. An isolated abnormal right-to-left relationship of either the atria or the ventricles is called *atrial or ventricular inversion*. In Figure 8–3,C, ventricular inversion or AV discor-

dance is shown. In this case the P axis is normal but the septal activation is reversed as it is in L-transposition of the great arteries (discussed later). Therefore, Q waves will be present in V4R through V6R but not in V5 or V6.

4. *Undifferentiated cardiac chambers* are often associated with complicated heart defects and unusual situs (situs ambiguous), as is seen in asplenia (Ivemark) syndrome or polysplenia syndrome (Fig 8–3,D). In these syndromes, owing to persistence of fetal bilaterality, the liver is large and transverse ("midline liver"). The cardiac apex is in the right side of the chest in about one half of the cases. These syndromes are usually associated with multiple intracardiac and extracardiac anomalies, making surgical correction difficult.

Example (Fig 8–4)

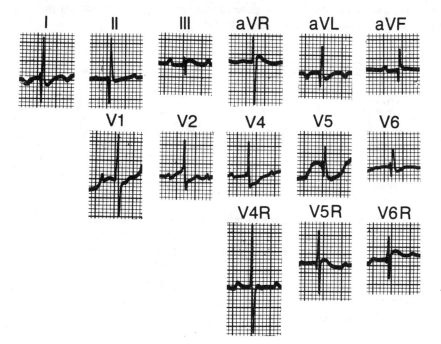

FIG 8–4.
Tracing from a 5-day-old infant with dextrocardia, ventricular septal defect, patent ductus arteriosus, and interrupted aortic arch.

In Figure 8–4, the P axis is around +120 degrees, suggesting that the sinus node is located on the left side (atrial situs inversus). No Q waves are seen in leads I and V6, where Q waves are normally seen. These two leads show, instead, small r waves, producing rsR′ patterns. Note the progressive decrease in the amplitude as one moves toward the V6 position. Definite Q waves are seen in V5R and V6R, suggesting that the left ventricle is located on the right rather than on the left. Other abnormalities in this tracing include prolonged PR interval (PR = 0.17) and upright T waves in V2 (which is analogous to V1 in a patient with dextrocardia). Flat or small T waves are not necessarily abnormal at this age. Therefore, the above ECG tracing suggests that the RA and RV are located on the left side of the LA and LV but in the right side of the chest. This infant had mirror-image dextrocardia with associated cardiac defects (this is an example of Fig 8–3,A).

Example (Fig 8–5)

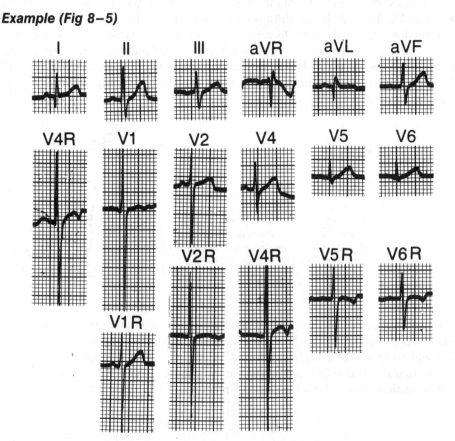

FIG 8–5.
Tracing from a 2-year-old child whose heart is located in the right side of the chest (revealed by x-ray films). He was asymptomatic and had abdominal situs solitus (stomach located on the left side and liver on the right).

In Figure 8–5, the P axis is 0 degrees, suggesting that the RA is on the right side of the LA (atrial situs solitus). Although the QRS deflections progressively decrease in amplitude toward V6, a definite Q wave is seen in V6, indicating that the LV is to the left of the RV. This is supported by the presence of Q waves in lead I and confirmed by the fact that no Q waves are seen in any of the right-sided precordial leads. In summary, this child had a normally formed heart that was rotated to the right because of hypoplasia of the right lung. This is an example of Figure 8–3,B (dextroversion).

Heart in the Left Side of the Chest

Abnormal chamber position can also be present in patients with levocardia.

1. In *patients with levocardia and abdominal situs inversus* the opposite of Figures 8–3,A and 8–3,B may occur.

2. *Congenitally corrected transposition (L-transposition) of the great arteries* is a condition in which the atria are located normally (the RA on the right side and the LA on the left side), but the ventricles are inverted, including the corresponding atrioventricular valves; that is, the RV is located on the left side and is connected to the LA through the tricuspid valve, and the LV is on the right side and is connected to the RA through the mitral valve (Fig 8–6). The great arteries are transposed, with the PA arising from the LV and the aorta from the RV (not shown in Fig 8–6). Although there is anatomical transposition of the great arteries, ventricular inversion permits the aorta to carry highly oxygenated blood, and the patient is not cyanotic. Oxygenated blood coming into the LA goes to the anatomical RV, through the tricuspid valve, and out the aorta. This is why the term "corrected" transposition has been used for this condition (Fig 8–6). This condition is described as atrial situs solitus, AV discordance, and ventriculoarterial discordance.

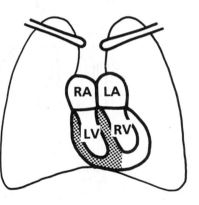

FIG 8–6.
Diagram of L-transposition of the great arteries. Note that the atria are situated in normal relation to one another (atrial situs solitus), but the ventricles are inverted. The septal depolarization proceeds leftward from the anatomical LV (right-sided ventricle), producing Q waves in the RPLs but no Q waves in the LPLs.

In congenitally corrected transposition, the P axis is normal (0 to +90 degrees). Reversed direction of ventricular septal activation produces Q waves in the right precordial leads (V4R, V1, etc.) and no Q waves in leads I, V5, and V6 (Fig 8–7). In addition to the intracardiac defects (ventricular septal defect, pulmonary stenosis) that may make them symptomatic early in life, these patients have a high incidence of progressive AV block.

Example (Fig 8–7)

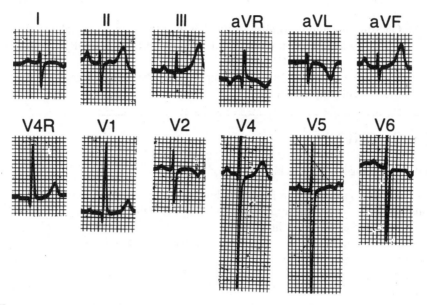

FIG 8–7.
Tracing from an 8-year-old cyanotic girl with L-transposition of the great arteries, ventricular septal defect, and severe pulmonary stenosis. The heart was in the left side of the chest.

In Fig 8–7, the P axis is +60 degrees, suggesting that the RA is on the right side. No Q waves are seen in leads I, V5, and V6. Instead the Q waves are seen in V4R and V1. This suggests that the LV is on the right side of the RV (ventricular inversion). Another abnormality seen in this tracing is severe RVH (or hypertrophy of the right and anteriorly located ventricle, the anatomical LV).

Single Ventricle

Normal Q waves (or the initial QRS vector) are produced primarily by ventricular septal depolarization. Therefore, abnormal Q waves are anticipated in cases of single ventricle where the ventricular septum is either absent or rudimentary.

Electrocardiographic findings in these cases are related to (1) the absence of normal septal depolarization, (2) the presence of only one ventricle, and (3) an abnormal conduction system.

1. An abnormal Q wave (or initial QRS vector) presents as one of the following:
   a. Absence of Q waves in all the precordial leads (seen in 60% of cases). The initial QRS vector is directed anteriorly and slightly to the left.
   b. Q waves are present in all the precordial leads (15% of cases). The initial QRS vector is directed posteriorly and slightly to the right.

   c. Q waves are present in the RPLs (V1 and V4R) but absent in the LPLs (V5 and V6) (seen in 25% of cases). The initial vector is directed leftward and posteriorly (see Fig 9–15).

2. The QRS morphology is similar throughout the precordial leads (abnormal R/S progression), since there is only one (functioning) ventricle. The QRS complex may assume either rS, RS, or QR patterns.
3. First- and second-degree AV blocks, supraventricular tachycardia, or WPW syndrome are frequently present.

REVIEW QUESTIONS

Answer the following questions either "true" or "false."

1. If the P axis is in the right lower quadrant (+90 to +180 degrees), the anatomical right atrium is likely to be on the right.   True   False
2. The presence of Q waves in V4R and V1 and the absence of Q waves in V5 and V6 may be seen in L-transposition of the great arteries or single ventricle.   True   False
3. If V5 and V6 show Q waves, the left ventricle is likely to be on the left (of the right ventricle).   True   False
4. In a patient with situs inversus totalis who is otherwise healthy, the P axis will be in the right lower quadrant (+90 to +180 degrees) and the Q wave will be seen in V5R and V6R.   True   False

Answers may be found on page 239.

CHAPTER 9

Systematic Approach

A systematic approach to interpretation of the ECG is essential. In this chapter some illustrative ECG tracings will be shown with narrative interpretations using a systematic approach. This chapter will also serve as an exercise for the readers if they cover the portion of narrative interpretation with a sheet of paper and work independently, in the space provided below each ECG tracing. Figures 9–1 and 9–2 serve as examples.

The following sequence is one of the many approaches that can be used:

1. Rhythm (sinus or nonsinus) by considering the P axis.
2. Heart rate (atrial and ventricular rates, if different).
3. The QRS axis, the T axis, and the QRS-T angle.
4. Intervals: PR, QRS, and QT.
5. The P wave amplitude and duration.
6. The QRS amplitude and the R/S ratio; also note abnormal Q waves.
7. ST segment and T wave abnormalities.

The report will contain the least chance of error if simple descriptive language is used and if it is confined to noting the duration, direction, morphology, and voltages of complexes. Making more precise anatomical and functional diagnoses should be left to the physician who has other information about the patient.

It is important for the physician interpreting the ECG to have the following information:

1. Patient's age.
2. Clinical diagnoses, cardiac and others.
3. Cardiovascular drugs.
4. Electrolyte imbalance and/or therapy.
5. Indication for ECG.
6. Previous ECG (where and when).

CASE 1

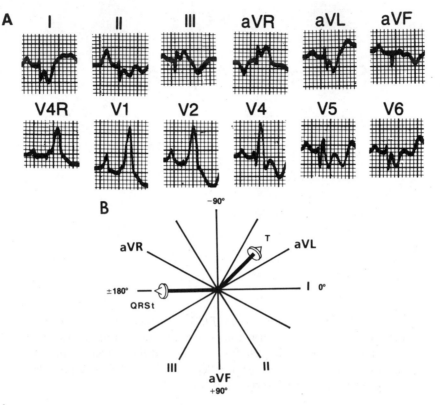

FIG 9–1.
Tracing from an 8-year-old boy with Ebstein's anomaly. The heart rate was 80 beats per minute in the original tracing.

Heart Rate _____80_____ (Atrial _____, Ventricular _____)
Rhythm ___Sinus___, P Amplitude ____4*____, P Duration ___0.1*___
PR ___0.17*___, QRS ___0.16*___, QT ___0.40*___
QRS Axis ___(t) + 180°___, T Axis ___−40°*___, QRS-T Angle ___>90°*___
Abnormal QRS Voltages and R/S Ratios:
   Abnormally large R/S ratios in V1 and V2.
ST-T Changes:
   T waves opposite to QRS complexes.
   *Denotes abnormalities
Interpretation:
   RAH, possible CAH, first-degree AV block, and RBBB.

Interpretation of Case 1

The rhythm is sinus. The P waves are tall, particularly in lead II (4 mm), and are relatively wide (0.10 second). The PR interval of 0.17 is slightly beyond the upper limits of normal (ULN) (0.16). The QRS duration (0.16 second) is markedly prolonged (ULN = 0.09 second), indicating a ventricular conduction disturbance. The slurring involves the terminal portion of the QRS complex and is directed to the right (wide S in I and V6) and anteriorly (wide R in V1 and V2), satisfying the criteria for RBBB. The terminal QRS axis (QRSt) is close to +180 degrees (see Fig 9–1). The QT interval is beyond the ULN in leads III and aVF (0.37); this is probably secondary to the wide QRS duration (RBBB). Although the R/S ratios in V1 and V2 are abnormally large, the diagnosis of ventricular hypertrophy is not justified in the presence of RBBB. The T axis is opposite to the major QRS force and outside the normal quadrant; this is secondary to RBBB. Abnormalities in this tracing include abnormally tall and relatively wide P waves, prolonged PR interval, and prolonged QRS duration with bizarre notching and terminal slurring that is directed to the right and anteriorly.

Interpretation: RAH, possible CAH, first-degree AV block, and RBBB.

CASE 2

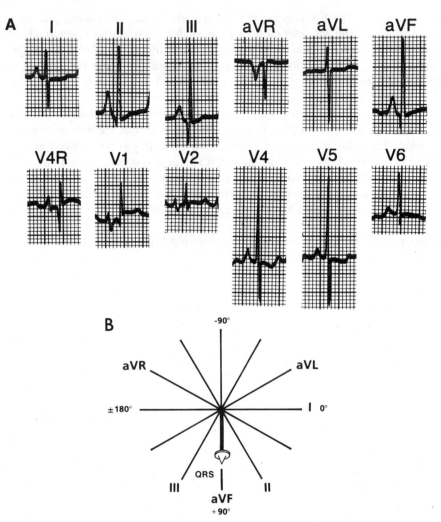

FIG 9–2.
Tracing from a 2-month-old boy with pulmonary atresia and a Blalock-Taussig shunt. He is receiving digoxin. The heart rate was 130 beats per minute in the original tracing.

Heart Rate ____*130*____ (Atrial _____ , Ventricular _____)
Rhythm ___*Sinus*___ , P Amplitude _____*5**_____ , P Duration ____*0.09**____
PR ___*0.12*___ , QRS ___*0.06*___ , QT _____
QRS Axis ___*+90°*___ , T Axis _*Low amplitude*_ , QRS-T Angle _____
Abnormal QRS Voltages and R/S Ratios:
   R in III (22) abnormally large.
   R in aVF (20) at the ULN.
ST-T Changes:
   ST segment shifts in V1, V5, and V6.
   *Denotes abnormalities
Interpretation:
   CAH, probable LVH, and probable digitalis effect.

Interpretation of Case 2

Sinus rhythm is present (the P axis is +60 degrees). The QRS axis is +90 degrees. The T axis and QT interval are not obtainable because of flat T waves in the limb leads. The PR interval (0.12) and the QRS duration (0.06) are normal. The P amplitude is abnormally large (6 mm in II), indicating RAH. The P duration is also relatively wide, 0.09 second, and the P waves are biphasic with prominent terminal negative deflection in V1, suggesting additional LAH. The R waves in lead III (22 mm) and aVF (20 mm) are slightly beyond and at the ULN (20 mm), respectively, indicating an abnormally strong downward force and probable LVH, considering that the precordial leads show left ventricular dominance. There are q waves in V4R and V1, in the absence of q waves in the LPLs, an abnormal finding. This raises the possibility of RVH as well. Other conditions associated with a q wave in the RPLs are ventricular inversion and single ventricle (see Chap. 3). ST segment shift (elevated in V1 and slightly depressed in V5) is present, but not necessarily abnormal. The ST and T changes may be due to digitalis. Shortening of the QTc is not possible to assess.

Interpretation: CAH, probable CVH, and probable digitalis effect.

CASE 3

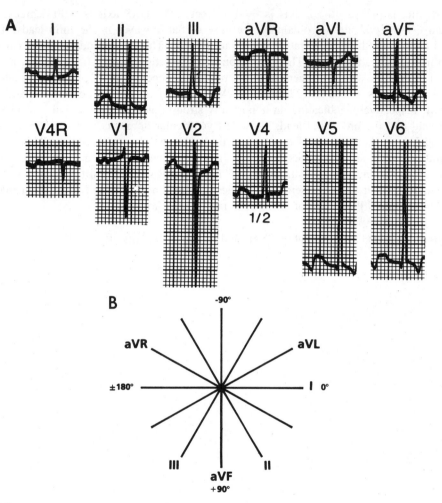

FIG 9–3.
Tracing from a 10-year-old boy who has had repeated attacks of rheumatic fever with severe aortic regurgitation. He is receiving digoxin. The heart rate was 120 beats per minute in the original tracing.

Heart Rate ____*120*____ (Atrial _____, Ventricular _____)
Rhythm _____, P Amplitude _____, P Duration _____
PR _____, QRS _____, QT _____
QRS Axis _____, T Axis _____, QRS-T Angle _____
Abnormal QRS Voltages and R/S Ratios:

ST-T Changes:

Interpretation:

Interpretation of Case 3

Although the P waves are not visible in most limb leads, they are upright in lead I and inverted in aVR (sinus rhythm). The P waves are also wide (0.13 second) (LAH). The PR interval also is long, being 0.28 second in leads II and aVR (first-degree AV block). The terminal positive portion of the T wave in aVF is the (positive) P wave. The QRS axis is +70 degrees and the T axis is around −60 degrees (the T wave is deepest in lead III), giving a wide QRS-T angle of more than 90 degrees, with the T axis in an abnormal quadrant. The QRS duration is 0.08. The QT interval is approximately 0.26, which is relatively short. Although the S in V2 and the R in V5 appear abnormally large, they are still within normal limits. The R in V6 (32 mm), however, is abnormally tall (ULN = 24). The R/S ratios are all normal. Abnormalities in this tracing are, therefore, prolonged PR interval, wide P waves, abnormally tall R in V6, abnormal T vector, wide QRS-T angle, and relatively short QT interval.

Interpretation: First-degree AV block, LAH, LVH with "strain," and probable digitalis effect.

CASE 4

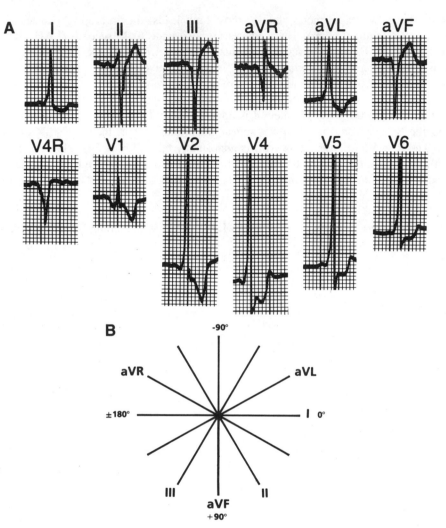

FIG 9–4.
Tracing from a 2-year-old boy whose VSD underwent spontaneous closure. He is asymptomatic, has no history of paroxysmal tachycardia, and is receiving no medication. The heart rate was 100 beats per minute in the original tracing.

Heart Rate ___*100*___ (Atrial _____, Ventricular _____)
Rhythm _____, P Amplitude _____, P Duration _____
PR _____, QRS _____, QT _____
QRS Axis _____, T Axis _____, QRS-T Angle _____
Abnormal QRS Voltages and R/S Ratios:

ST-T Changes:

Interpretation:

Interpretation of Case 4

A small P wave is present in front of each QRS complex, and the P axis indicates sinus rhythm. The P wave amplitude and duration are normal. The QRS axis is abnormal (−60 degrees) and the T axis is +100 degrees, which gives a wide QRS-T angle (160 degrees). The most striking abnormalities are a short PR interval (0.08) (LLN = 0.08) and a wide QRS duration (0.11) (ULN = 0.07). On closer inspection we see delta waves in most of the leads. ST segments and T waves are shifted opposite to the direction of the QRS vector, which results in a wide QRS-T angle. (This is not uncommon in ventricular conduction disturbances.) These findings are compatible with Wolff-Parkinson-White syndrome. The general sequence of the delta wave and the major part of the QRS are directed to the left and posteriorly, indicating a right ventricular origin of the preexcitation. Although some QRS deflections are abnormally large, diagnosis of ventricular hypertrophy cannot be made when WPW syndrome is present.

Interpretation: Wolff-Parkinson-White syndrome.

CASE 5

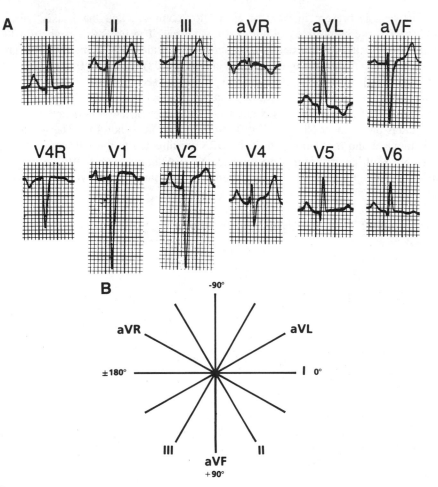

FIG 9–5.
Tracing from a 7-year-old boy with tricuspid atresia for which a Blalock-Taussig shunt surgery was performed. The heart rate was 75 beats per minute in the original tracing.

Heart Rate ___75___ (Atrial _____, Ventricular _____)
Rhythm _____, P Amplitude _____, P Duration _____
PR _____, QRS _____, QT _____
QRS Axis _____, T Axis _____, QRS-T Angle _____
Abnormal QRS Voltages and R/S Ratios:

ST-T Changes:

Interpretation:

Interpretation of Case 5

Sinus rhythm is present (with the P axis of +15 degrees). The P amplitude is greater than 3 mm in lead I (RAH), and the P duration is 0.11 second, which is abnormally long (LAH). The P wave in lead I has characteristic notching of CAH. The PR interval of 0.16 second is normal for the heart rate and age of the patient. The QRS duration (0.08) is at the ULN, and the QT interval (0.36) is normal. The QRS axis is −60 degrees (left anterior hemiblock or superior QRS axis), and the T axis is approximately +80 degrees, with the QRS-T angle of 150 degrees, but the T axis is in the normal quadrant. The R wave in aVL (17 mm) and the S wave in V4R (13 mm) are greater than the ULN, suggesting abnormal leftward force. The R/S ratio in V1 is smaller than the LLN, suggesting LVH.

Interpretation: Superior QRS axis (left anterior hemiblock), CAH, and LVH.

CASE 6

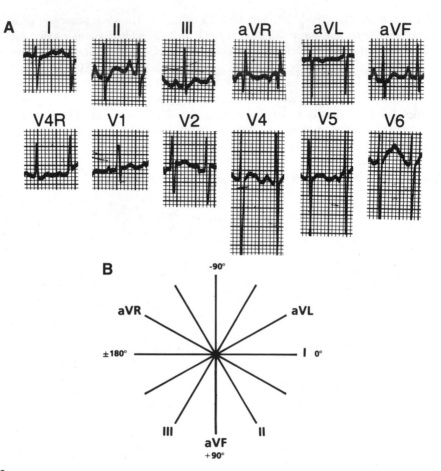

FIG 9–6.
Tracing from a 6-day-old male infant with ᴅ-transposition of the great arteries and small VSD.

Heart Rate _____ (Atrial _____ , Ventricular _____)
Rhythm _____ , P Amplitude _____ , P Duration _____
PR _____ , QRS _____ , QT _____
QRS Axis _____ , T Axis _____ , QRS-T Angle _____
Abnormal QRS Voltages and R/S Ratios:

ST-T Changes:

Interpretation:

Interpretation of Case 6

Sinus rhythm is present with a heart rate of 160 beats per minute. The P wave amplitude of 3 mm in lead II is abnormally tall. The QRS axis is +140 degrees and the T axis is +70 degrees. The QRS-T angle of this magnitude (70 degrees) is not abnormal in a newborn infant, considering that the T vector is in the normal quadrant (0 to +90 degrees). The PR interval (0.11), the QRS duration (0.05), and the QT interval (0.22) are all within normal limits. The S waves in V5 and V6 are deeper than the ULN, suggesting abnormal rightward force (RVH). The abnormal rightward force is also reflected in deep S waves (10 mm) in lead I (at the ULN). The upright T wave in V1 is also abnormal for the patient's age, consistent with RVH.

Interpretation: RAH and RVH.

CASE 7

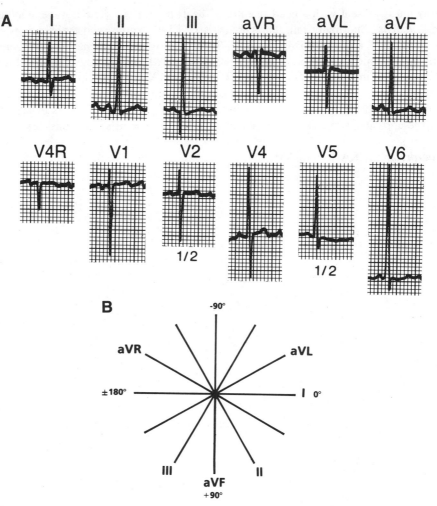

FIG 9–7.

Tracing from a 3-month-old infant with clinical diagnosis of endocardial fibroelastosis. The heart rate was 145 beats per minute in the original tracing.

Heart Rate ____145____ (Atrial _____, Ventricular _____)

Rhythm _____, P Amplitude _____, P Duration _____

PR _____, QRS _____, QT _____

QRS Axis _____, T Axis _____, QRS-T Angle _____

Abnormal QRS Voltages and R/S Ratios:

ST-T Changes:

Interpretation:

Interpretation of Case 7

Sinus rhythm is present, since P waves are upright in leads I and aVF, as well as in lead II. The P amplitude and duration are within normal limits. The PR interval of 0.10 is relatively short, but not abnormally so (see Chap. 3). No delta wave is present. The QRS duration (0.06) and the QT interval (0.36) are both normal. The QRS axis is +70 degrees and the T axis +60 degrees, with normal QRS-T angle. The R wave in lead II (20 mm) is at the ULN and that in aVF is near the ULN. The R waves in V5 (32 mm) and V6 (30 mm) are abnormally tall, indicating abnormal leftward force. The S wave in V1 (18 mm) is also at the ULN, but that in V2 is not too deep. Therefore, the QRS voltages in this tracing show abnormally strong leftward force with near abnormal forces inferiorly and posteriorly, justifying the diagnosis of LVH.

Interpretation: LVH.

CASE 8

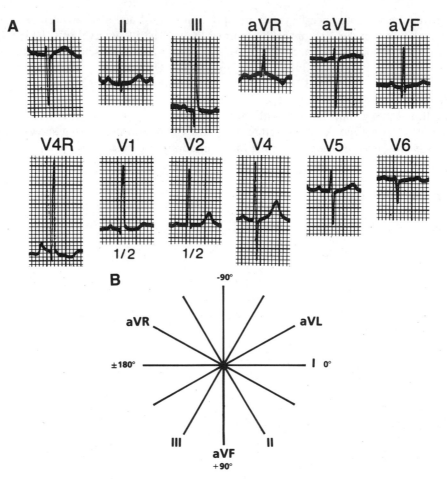

FIG 9–8.
Tracing from a 4-year-old girl with complete transposition of the great arteries for which the Mustard operation was performed. The heart rate was 120 beats per minute in the original tracing.

Heart Rate ____*120*____ (Atrial _____ , Ventricular _____)
Rhythm _____ , P Amplitude _____ , P Duration _____
PR _____ , QRS _____ , QT _____
QRS Axis _____ , T Axis _____ , QRS-T Angle _____
Abnormal QRS Voltages and R/S Ratios:

ST-T Changes:

Interpretation:

Interpretation of Case 8

The rhythm is sinus since P waves are upright in leads II and aVF and are inverted in aVR. The P amplitude and duration are normal. The PR interval (0.14), the QRS duration (0.05), and the QT interval (0.30) are all within normal limits. The QRS axis is about +130 degrees (RAD), and the T axis +40 degrees. The QRS-T angle is wide (90 degrees), but the T axis remains in the normal quadrant (0 to +90 degrees). The S waves in lead I (13 mm) and in V6 (6 mm) are abnormally deep. The R waves in V4R (24 mm) and V1 (33 mm) are abnormal, all indicating RVH. The R/S ratios are also abnormal in V1, V2, and V6, in favor of the RVH. The above findings are indicative of RVH, with a wide QRS-T angle but with the T axis remaining in the normal quadrant (possible "strain" pattern). There are q waves in V4R and V1, also suggestive of RVH.

Interpretation: RVH with possible "strain."

CASE 9

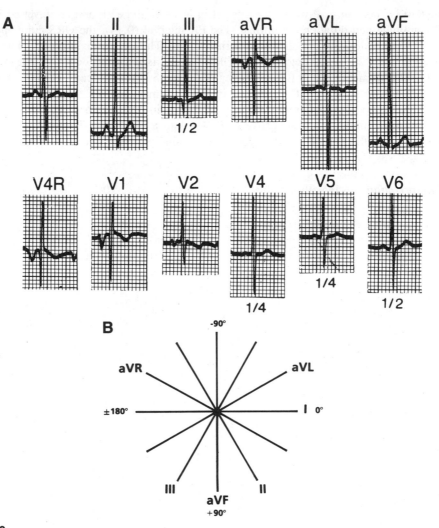

FIG 9–9.
Tracing from a 5-week-old male infant with persistent truncus arteriosus, type I. The heart rate was 120 beats per minute in the original tracing.

Heart Rate ____*120*____ (Atrial _____, Ventricular _____)
Rhythm _____, P Amplitude _____, P Duration _____
PR _____, QRS _____, QT _____
QRS Axis _____, T Axis _____, QRS-T Angle _____
Abnormal QRS Voltages and R/S Ratios:

ST-T Changes:

Interpretation:

Interpretation of Case 9

The P waves in this tracing indicate sinus rhythm. The PR interval is 0.10. The QRS axis is about +85 degrees and the T axis is +80 degrees. The QRS duration (0.06) and the QT interval (0.24) are normal. The P waves are peaked (2.5 mm) but not quite abnormal (ULN = 2.5 mm). The P in V1 has an initial, small, upright deflection followed by a deep, terminal, negative deflection with total P wave duration of 0.08, indicating probable LAH, in spite of the duration being WNL (a P duration of 0.08 second and longer is abnormal in infants less than 12 months of age; in children, the P duration of 0.1 second and longer is abnormal). There are strong downward (tall R in II, III, and aVF) and leftward (tall R in I, V5, and V6) as well as rightward (tall R in V4R and deep S in I, V5, and V6) forces, indicating combined ventricular hypertrophy. Note one-half standardization in III and V6 and one-fourth standardization in V4 and V5.

Interpretation: CVH and probable LAH.

CASE 10

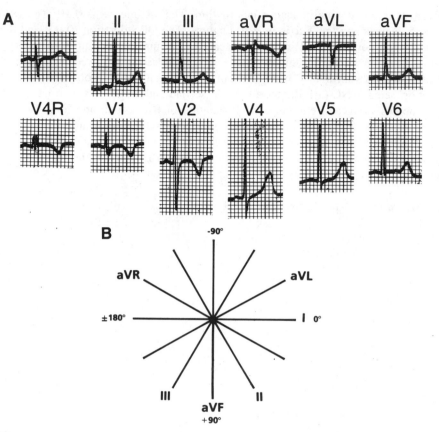

FIG 9-10.
Tracing from a 5-year-old asymptomatic girl who had heart murmur on routine physical examination. The heart rate was 80 beats per minute in the original tracing.

Heart Rate ____*80*____ (Atrial _____ , Ventricular _____)
Rhythm _____ , P Amplitude _____ , P Duration _____
PR _____ , QRS _____ , QT _____
QRS Axis _____ , T Axis _____ , QRS-T Angle _____
Abnormal QRS Voltages and R/S Ratios:

ST-T Changes:

Interpretation:

Interpretation of Case 10

Sinus rhythm is present with the P axis of +30 degrees. The QRS axis is +90 degrees and the T axis +60 degrees, with normal QRS-T angle. The PR interval (0.11), the QRS duration (0.06), and the QT interval (0.34) are all WNL. There is an rsr′ pattern in V4R and rss′ pattern in V1. This kind of rsr′ pattern in the RPLs is a normal finding in children as long as the QRS duration is normal. A similar finding is shown as an example of a normal 2-month-old infant in Figure 2−3. A little notching in the downstroke of R waves in lead III of this tracing and in V1 of Figure 2−3 is also a normal finding.

Interpretation: Normal ECG.

CASE 11

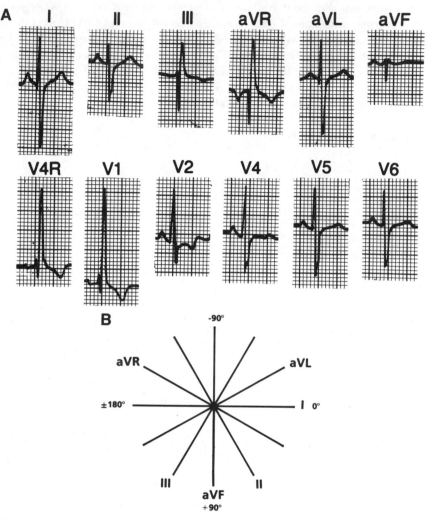

FIG 9–11.

Tracing from a 12-year-old girl who had Down's Syndrome, severe tetralogy of Fallot, and endocardial cushion defect. An aortic-right pulmonary artery shunt (Waterston procedure) was performed early in life. The heart rate was 70 beats per minute in the original tracing.

Heart Rate _____*70*_____ (Atrial _____, Ventricular _____)

Rhythm _____, P Amplitude _____, P Duration _____

PR _____, QRS _____, QT _____

QRS Axis _____, T Axis _____, QRS-T Angle _____

Abnormal QRS Voltages and R/S Ratios:

ST-T Changes:

Interpretation:

Interpretation of Case 11

Sinus rhythm is present with the P axis of +30 degrees. The P amplitude and duration are normal. The PR interval (0.14) and the QT interval (0.36) are normal for the heart rate. There is a slight terminal slurring of the QRS complex, but the QRS duration (0.09) is within normal limits (ULN = 0.10). Therefore, ventricular conduction disturbance is not present. The QRS axis cannot easily be plotted. It requires the use of two-vector plot (see Chap. 1). The initial QRS vector (QRSi) is −20 degrees, and the terminal vector (QRSt) is approximately +180 degrees. In other words, there are two strong opposing vectors, initially leftward and terminally rightward. If one had used one-vector plot, the QRS axis would have been plotted to be −100 degrees, to which the QRS vector is very weak. The T axis is +10 degrees. The rightward QRS voltages are abnormal, manifested by deep S waves in lead I (16 mm) and V6 (10 mm), and tall R waves in aVR (13 mm), V4R (21 mm), and V1 (25 mm), all beyond the ULN (severe RVH). The R/S ratios in V1, V2, and V6 are all abnormal, suggesting RVH.

Interpretation: Severe RVH. Superior QRS axis.

CASE 12

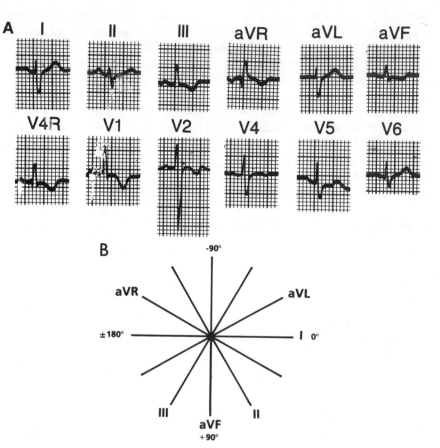

FIG 9–12.

Tracing from a 4-year-old girl with secundum type atrial septal defect. The heart rate was 70 beats per minute.

Heart Rate _____*70*_____ (Atrial _____, Ventricular _____)
Rhythm _____, P Amplitude _____, P Duration _____
PR _____, QRS _____, QT _____
QRS Axis _____, T Axis _____, QRS-T Angle _____
Abnormal QRS Voltages and R/S Ratios:

ST-T Changes:

Interpretation:

Interpretation of Case 12

Sinus rhythm is present. The P amplitude and duration are normal. The PR interval (0.14) and the QT interval (0.32) are both normal for the heart rate. There is slight terminal slurring of the QRS complex (wide S waves in lead I, aVL, V5 and V6, and wide R waves in aVR and V1), and the QRS duration (0.09) is slightly beyond the ULN (0.08 in a 4-year-old child), indicating RBBB. The QRS axis is +130 degrees, RAD for age. The T axis is 0 degrees. The QRS voltages are all within normal limits. The only abnormality is the R/S ratio in V1 (greater than 10) which is beyond the ULN (2), suggesting only possible RVH, especially in the presence of RBBB. A common ECG finding in children with ASD is RAD and rsR′ pattern in V1, although this patient does not have the classic rsR′ pattern in V1.

Interpretation: RAD, RBBB, and possible RVH.

CASE 13

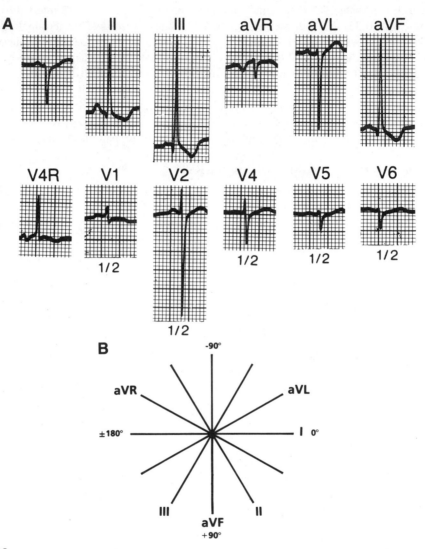

FIG 9–13.
Tracing from a 4-year-old boy with severe pulmonary stenosis. He is receiving digoxin. The heart rate was 80 beats per minute in the original tracing.

Heart Rate _____*80*_____ (Atrial _____, Ventricular _____)

Rhythm _____, P Amplitude _____, P Duration _____

PR _____, QRS _____, QT _____

QRS Axis _____, T Axis _____, QRS-T Angle _____

Abnormal QRS Voltages and R/S Ratios:

ST-T Changes:

Interpretation:

Interpretation of Case 13

Sinus rhythm is present, judging from the P axis. The P amplitude and duration are normal. The PR interval (0.14) and the QRS duration (0.07) are within normal limits. The QT interval (0.23) is relatively short, suggesting digitalis effect. The QRS axis is +110 degrees. The T axis is −80 degrees with resulting wide QRS-T angle (190 degrees). The T axis is outside the normal range, suggesting a "strain" pattern rather than digitalis effect. Digitalis does not change the T axis or QRS-T angle (see Chap. 6, digitalis effect). The R waves in leads III (29 mm) and aVF (24 mm) are abnormally large, indicating abnormal inferior force. The R in V4R (11 mm) and the S in I (10 mm) are beyond the ULN, indicating abnormal rightward force. The S in V2 (54 mm, note one-half standardization) is abnormally deep (ULN = 38). This deep S in V2 probably represents right ventricular force (rather than left ventricular force) which is directed markedly rightward and not anteriorly. V2 is not a pure Z-axis lead and can respond with a deep S caused by markedly rightward forces.

Interpretation: RVH with "strain" and digitalis effect.

CASE 14

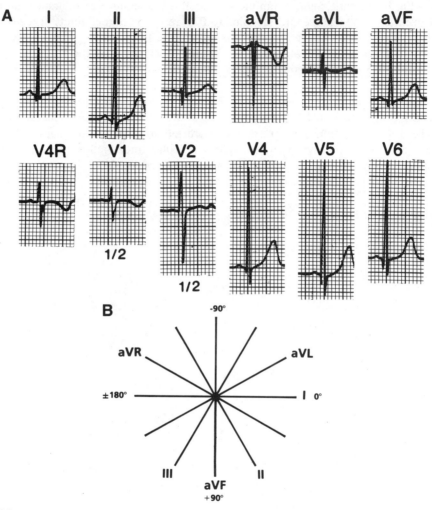

FIG 9–14.
Tracing from a healthy 8-year-old boy. The heart rate was 84 beats per minute in the original tracing.

Heart Rate _____*84*_____ (Atrial _____, Ventricular _____)
Rhythm _____, P Amplitude _____, P Duration _____
PR _____, QRS _____, QT _____
QRS Axis _____, T Axis _____, QRS-T Angle _____
Abnormal QRS Voltages and R/S Ratios:

ST-T Changes:

Interpretation:

Interpretation of Case 14

The rhythm is sinus. The P wave amplitude and duration are normal. The PR interval (0.12), the QRS duration (0.07), and the QT interval (0.38) are all within normal limits. The QRS axis is +60 degrees and the T axis is +50 degrees with a QRS-T angle of 10 degrees. The QRS voltages are normal except for the R wave of V6 (26 mm), which is slightly beyond the ULN (24 mm). The R in V5 is WNL. No ST-T changes are present. The amplitudes of Q and T waves are normal in V5 and V6. In the absence of other abnormalities, an R wave amplitude in V6 slightly beyond the ULN is a weak criterion of LVH (see Chap. 4) and is often due to imprecise location of the V6 electrode. In fact, a repeated ECG on this boy showed normal R voltage in V6.

Interpretation: Normal ECG.

CASE 15

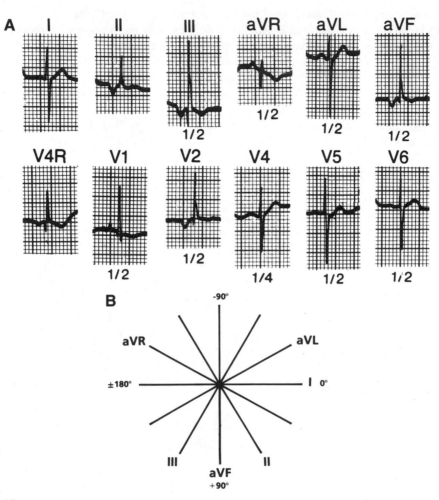

FIG 9–15.

Tracing from a 3-month-old male infant with single ventricle and single atrium. The heart rate was 130 beats per minute in the original tracing.

Heart Rate ____*130*____ (Atrial _____, Ventricular _____)
Rhythm _____, P Amplitude _____, P Duration _____
PR _____, QRS _____, QT _____
QRS Axis _____, T Axis _____, QRS-T Angle _____
Abnormal QRS Voltages and R/S Ratios:

ST-T Changes:

Interpretation:

Interpretation of Case 15

Although there are P waves in front of each QRS complex, the rhythm is not sinus, because the P axis is not in the normal quadrant. The P axis is −90 degrees, directed superiorly, suggesting an abnormal rhythm originating somewhere in the lower part of the atrial mass (low atrial rhythm, or "coronary sinus rhythm"). The P amplitude is 2.5 mm (WNL). The PR interval (0.11) and the QT interval (0.26) are within normal limits. The QRS duration (0.05) is normal. The QRS axis is +110 degrees and the T axis −10 degrees, with the QRS-T angle of 120 degrees. The S waves in lead I (11 mm), V5 (25 mm), V6 (22 mm), and the R wave in V2 (22 mm) are all beyond the ULN (abnormal rightward forces). The leftward force (R in V6) is generous but within normal limits. The abnormal rightward QRS forces are indicative of RVH, and abnormal inferior force might be an indication of additional LVH. There are q waves in V4R, V1, and V2, a common finding in patients with single ventricle (see Chap. 8). The R/S ratio in V6 is smaller than the LLN, again suggestive of RVH.

Interpretation: Low atrial rhythm, RVH, and possible additional LVH.

CASE 16

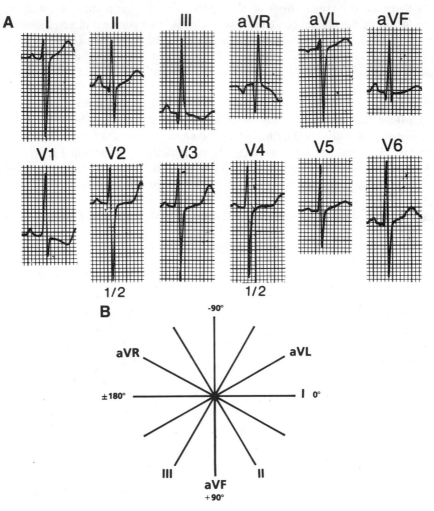

FIG 9–16.
Tracing from an 11-year-old child with cor pulmonale. The heart rate was 60 beats per minute in the original tracing.

Heart Rate _____60_____ (Atrial _____, Ventricular _____)
Rhythm _____, P Amplitude _____, P Duration _____
PR _____, QRS _____, QT _____
QRS Axis _____, T Axis _____, QRS-T Angle _____
Abnormal QRS Voltages and R/S Ratios:

ST-T Changes:

Interpretation:

Interpretation of Case 16

The rhythm is sinus. The P amplitude is 3 mm in II (RAH), but the P duration is normal. The PR interval (0.15) and the QT interval (0.40) are within normal limits. The QRS duration (0.09) is at the ULN. The QRS axis is +140 degrees, and the T axis is +15 degrees, with a resulting QRS-T angle of 125 degrees, but the T axis is in the normal quadrant. The S waves in I (20 mm) and V6 (14 mm) and the R waves in aVR (13 mm) are abnormally large (abnormal rightward force). The R wave in V1 (16 mm, right and anterior force) is at the ULN. The S wave in V2 (40 mm) is at the ULN. This S wave in V2 probably represents right ventricular force rather than left ventricular force, considering the right axis deviation of +140 degrees (see Chap. 1, horizontal reference system). The R/S ratio in V1 (3.0) is beyond the ULN (1.0), and that in V6 (1.0) is smaller than the LLN (4.0), again indicating abnormal RV force. The diagnosis of RVH is based on these findings. Although the T axis is in the normal quadrant, the diagnosis of RVH with possible "strain" is warranted by the abnormally wide QRS-T angle (125 degrees).

Interpretation: RVH with possible "strain," and RAH.

CASE 17

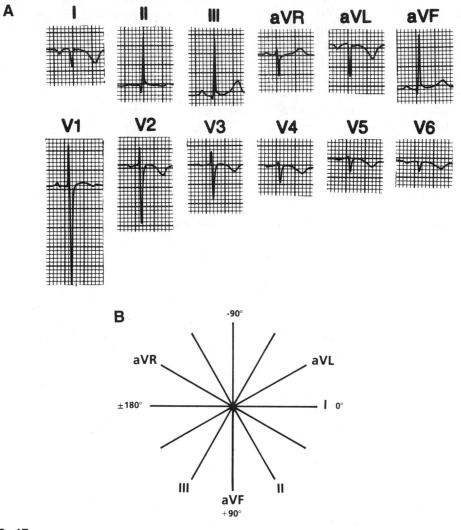

FIG 9–17.
Tracing from a 14-year-old child with dextrocardia. The heart rate was 76 beats per minute in the original tracing. *(Continued.)*

Heart Rate _____*76*_____ (Atrial _____, Ventricular _____)
Rhythm _____, P Amplitude _____, P Duration _____
PR _____, QRS _____, QT _____
QRS Axis _____, T Axis _____, QRS-T Angle _____
Abnormal QRS Voltages and R/S Ratios:

ST-T Changes:

Interpretation:

Interpretation of Case 17

The P axis is in the right lower quadrant (about +150 degrees, because the P wave is flat in lead II). The QRS axis is about +110 degrees and the T axis +150 degrees. This raises the possibility of situs inversus of the atria (seen in mirror-image dextrocardia) or incorrectly placed right and left arm electrodes. The precordial leads obtained on the left chest (shown in Fig 9–17) are also characteristic of the heart in the right chest; there is a progressive decrease in the amplitude of the QRS as one moves from V2 toward V6. The PR interval (0.16), QRS duration (0.07), and QT interval (0.36) are all within normal limits. The QRS voltages in V1 (which would be V2 in a patient with dextrocardia) are also within normal limit. This is later confirmed by a repeat ECG with right-sided precordial leads (Fig 9–17,C). V1R and V2R, etc., are obtained with chest electrodes in the mirror-image positions of V1 and V2, etc. There is a Q wave in V6R, indicating the anatomic LV is in the right lateral position or in the mirror-image position of normal LV. The QRS voltage in V6R (28 mm) is beyond the ULN, but other leads do not show abnormal forces in this direction; it is possibly factitious.

Interpretation: ECG compatible with mirror-image dextrocardia. Otherwise normal ECG.

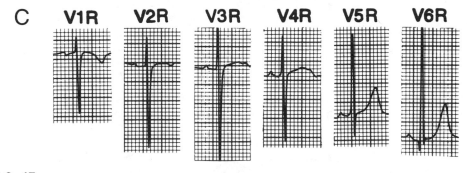

FIG 9–17.
C, precordial leads obtained from the right chest of patient in Case 17.

CASE 18

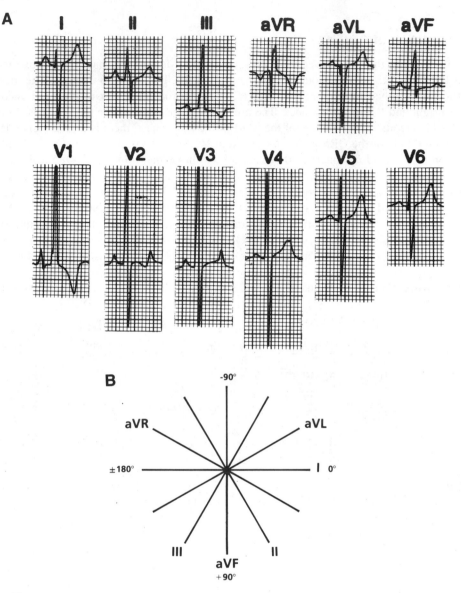

FIG 9–18.

Tracing from a 9-year-old child with tetralogy of Fallot with pulmonary atresia, hypoplasia of the left pulmonary artery, and extensive bronchial collaterals to the right lung. The heart rate was 92 beats per minute in the original tracing.

Heart Rate ____92____ (Atrial _____ , Ventricular _____)
Rhythm _____ , P Amplitude _____ , P Duration _____
PR _____ , QRS _____ , QT _____
QRS Axis _____ , T Axis _____ , QRS-T Angle _____
Abnormal QRS Voltages and R/S Ratios:

ST-T Changes:

Interpretation:

Interpretation of Case 18

The rhythm is sinus (with the P axis of +50 degrees). The QRS axis is +130 degrees, and the T axis +20 degrees. Although the QRS-T angle is wide (110 degrees), the T axis remains in the normal quadrant. The P wave is 3 mm in lead II (RAH), but its duration is not prolonged. The PR interval is normal (0.14). The QRS complex shows a terminal slurring directed to the right (slurred S in I and V6; slurred R in aVR and V1), but the QRS duration is not prolonged, being at the ULN. The right and anterior forces (S in I, V5, and V6, and R in aVR, V1, and V2) are abnormal, suggesting RVH. Although the QRS shows terminal slurring, suggesting RBBB, the QRS duration is within normal limits, a finding against that diagnosis. Rather, the abnormal QRS voltages favor the diagnosis of RVH. The presence of RAH strengthens the diagnosis of RVH.

Interpretation: Probable RVH, RAH.

CASE 19

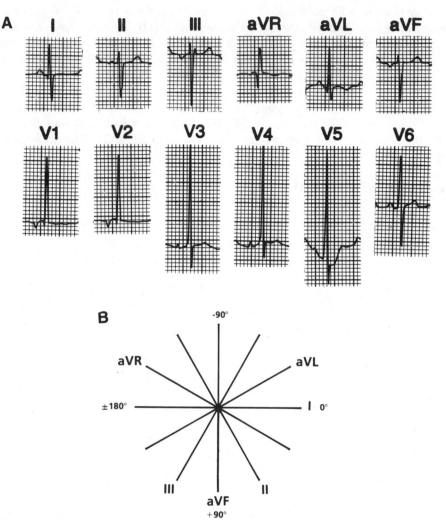

FIG 9–19.

Tracing from a 1-week-old neonate with mild cyanosis and a midline liver. The heart rate was 130 beats per minute in the original tracing.

Heart Rate _____130_____ (Atrial _____, Ventricular _____)

Rhythm _____, P Amplitude _____, P Duration _____

PR _____, QRS _____, QT _____

QRS Axis _____, T Axis _____, QRS-T Angle _____

Abnormal QRS Voltages and R/S Ratios:

ST-T Changes:

Interpretation:

Interpretation of Case 19

The P axis is in the left upper quadrant (−45 degrees), the wrong quadrant for sinus rhythm (ectopic low atrial rhythm). The QRS axis (−80 degrees) is also in the same quadrant (superior QRS axis). The T axis is +90 degrees. The PR interval looks relatively short (0.01), but is probably within normal limits. The QRS duration is 0.07 (at the ULN), and the QT interval (0.27) is normal. The P amplitude and duration are normal. There are pure R waves with q waves in V1 and V2 (RVH). The abnormally deep S wave in V6 (abnormal rightward force) is also noteworthy. A large R wave in V5 is at the ULN, suggesting additional LVH, confirmed by an R in aVL that is greater than normal. This infant is most likely to have polysplenia syndrome. Infants with polysplenia syndrome have an ectopic atrial pacemaker due to the absence of a sinus node (secondary to bilateral left atria), and superior QRS axis because of endocardial cushion defect, a constant component of the syndrome.

Interpretation: Ectopic atrial rhythm, superior QRS axis, RVH, probably additional LVH.

CASE 20

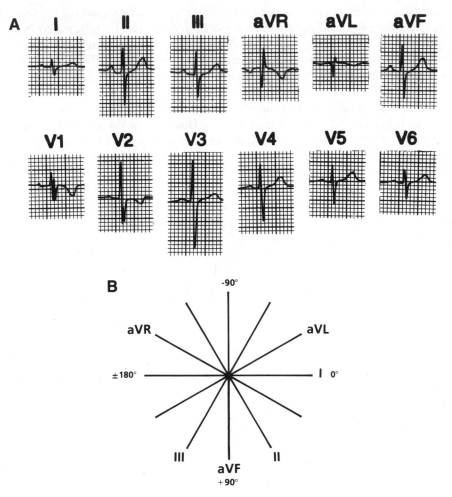

FIG 9–20.
Tracing from a 4-year-old child. The heart rate was 100 beats per minute in the original tracing.

Heart Rate ____*100*____ (Atrial _____, Ventricular _____)
Rhythm _____, P Amplitude _____, P Duration _____
PR _____, QRS _____, QT _____
QRS Axis _____, T Axis _____, QRS-T Angle _____
Abnormal QRS Voltages and R/S Ratios:

ST-T Changes:

Interpretation:

Interpretation of Case 20

Sinus rhythm is present with the P axis of +70 degrees. There are equiphasic QRS complexes in most limb leads, making it difficult to plot the QRS axis in the usual manner. One needs to use two-vector plot, by dividing the QRS complex into the initial and terminal portions. The initial QRS axis (QRSi) is +75 degrees (derived from the initial QRS amplitude of +2 mm in lead I and that of +7 mm in aVF). The terminal QRS vector (QRSt) is −105 degrees (derived from the terminal amplitude of −2 mm in lead I and that of −7 mm in aVF). The T axis is +75 degrees. The P amplitude and duration are normal. The PR interval is 0.16 (at the ULN). The QRS duration is 0.08 (at the ULN) without terminal slurring. The QRS voltages are all within normal limits in the limb leads and precordial leads. The rsr's' in V1 and the notched S in V2 are not abnormal at this age, provided the QRS duration is not prolonged.

Interpretation: ECG within normal limits.

CHAPTER 10

Analysis of Arrhythmias and Atrioventricular Conduction Disturbances

As more and more physicians are involved in the care of sick patients in intensive care units or in emergency rooms, the ability to make correct diagnosis of rhythm disturbances has become essential for a wider range of physicians. In Chapter 7, characteristics of basic arrhythmias and AV conduction disturbances were presented using simple drawings of the disturbances. In this chapter, readers will have an opportunity to interpret actual rhythm strips on their own.

There are different ways of approaching arrhythmias; the choice depends upon the level of undertanding of the reader. Many books approach rhythm disturbances according to the abnormal mechanism underlying the disorders, starting with P waves and following rather complex diagrams. We believe this approach too cumbersome and difficult for beginners since the answer must be anticipated in order to even begin the analysis. We have found it easier for many to analyze starting with the *rate* and *regularity* (the rhythm method), to narrow down the possibilities (Table 10–1).

When one uses the rhythm method, one starts with inspection of the overall rhythm strip and asks the following questions:

Is the rhythm *regular?*

If so, is the *rate* normal, rapid, or slow?

If the rhythm is *irregular* (arrhythmia), is there pattern of irregularity to the rhythm *(regularly irregular),* or is it totally irregular *(irregularly irregular)?*

If only a beat or two interrupt the regularity, is the abnormal beat *premature* (ectopic beat) or is there a *long pause?*

TABLE 10-1.

The Rhythm Method

I. Regular rhythm
  A. Normal rate
    1. Regular sinus rhythm
    2. Nonsinus rhythm
      Ectopic atrial pacemaker ("coronary sinus" rhythm)
      Accelerated AV nodal rhythm
      2:1 AV block with sinus or atrial tachycardia
      Implanted ventricular pacemaker
  B. Rapid rate
    Sinus tachycardia
    Supraventricular tachycardia
      (Ectopic atrial tachycardia, reciprocating AV tachycardia,
      and nodal [junctional] tachycardia)
    Ventricular tachycardia
  C. Slow rate
    Sinus bradycardia
    AV nodal rhythm with SA block or complete AV block
    Idioventricular rhythm with SA block or complete AV block
II. Irregular rhythm
  A. Regular arrhythmias
    (Regularly irregular)
    Sinus arrhythmia
    Wenckebach (Mobitz type I)
    Bigeminy (atrial, AV nodal, ventricular)
    Trigeminy (atrial, AV nodal, ventricular)
  B. Irregular arrhythmias
    (Irregularly irregular)
    Atrial fibrillation
    Atrial flutter with variable AV block
    Ventricular fibrillation
  C. *Single* or *infrequent* irregularity
    Premature beats (atrial, AV nodal, ventricular)
    AV dissociation with interference
    Second-degree AV block (Mobitz type II)
III. Long pause
  Sinus pause or arrest
  Complete AV block with no escape

Another method that is a little more mechanism-oriented uses the relationship of the P wave to the QRS complex (the P-wave method, Table 10-2). In this approach, the first step is to decide whether sinus rhythm is present or not. If sinus rhythm is present, one then determines which of the sinus rhythms it is—for example, sinus bradycardia or sinus arrhythmia. If the rhythm is not sinus, the presence or absence of P waves and the number and morphologic features of P waves are noted. When the P wave is irregularly related to the QRS complex, one should mark P waves across the rhythm strip (see the "walk out" method, below). Table 10-2 is then used to narrow down the possibilities. In pinpointing the diagnosis, the QRS duration is often helpful; a normal QRS duration rules out ventricular arrhythmias.

TABLE 10–2.

The P-Wave Method

I. Sinus rhythm*:	Regular sinus rhythm	
	Sinus tachycardia	
	Sinus bradycardia	
	Sinus arrhythmia	
	Sinus pause or arrest	

II. Nonsinus rhythm:
  A. Abnormal shape of P waves (abnormal P-axis):

Single or infrequent beats:	PAC (premature atrial contraction)
Gradual changes:	Wandering atrial pacemaker
Constant abnormality:	Ectopic atrial pacemaker rhythm
	Atrial situs inversus
	Incorrectly placed arm leads
	Nodal rhythm with retrogradely conducted P waves
	Reciprocating AV tachycardia (SVT)

  B. More than one P for each QRS:

1. Fast P rate:	Ectopic atrial tachycardia (240 ± 40) with 2° AV block
	Atrial flutter (300 ± 50) with 2° AV block
	Atrial fibrillation (400 ± 50) with 2° AV block
2. Normal P rate:	Second-degree AV block
	(Mobitz types I and II, 2:1 or higher blocks)
	Complete AV block

  C. Absent P waves:

1. Single or infrequent absence:	SA block with nodal escape
	Nodal premature beats
	Premature ventricular contraction

    2. Constantly "absent" P (may be buried in T wave):

Nodal rhythm
Accelerated nodal rhythm
Nodal, atrial or reciprocating tachycardia (SVT)
Atrial fibrillation
Idioventricular rhythm
Ventricular tachycardia

*Includes first-degree AV block and ventricular conduction disturbances (bundle branch block, Wolff-Parkinson-White syndrome, etc.).

Since P waves are more reliably regular than other ECG waves, one identifies the P waves and maps out the P waves across the rhythm strip (the "walk out" method). This is done by locating two P waves in a row someplace in the strip and marking them on a piece of paper or setting dividers at that interval. The paper is advanced so that only one of the marks is on one of the P waves of the pair and marks where a P wave might be hidden. By continuing this process, one may unmask P waves hidden in other waves such as QRS complexes or T waves (Fig 10–1).

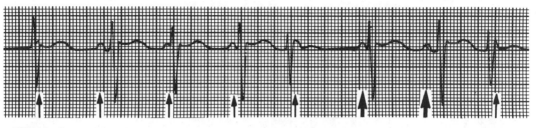

FIG 10–1.
The "walk out" method of identifying P waves. From inspection of the rhythm strip, it is clear that there are two P waves in a row toward the end of the strip (marked by *thicker arrows*). The measured PP interval is marched forward and backward, identifying P waves shown by the *thinner arrows*. Note that two P waves hidden in the first and the last QRS complexes are now uncovered. In addition to uncovering hidden P waves, this method can be used to distinguish artifacts from potential P waves.

One may use either one or both methods described above to narrow down the possibilities. One should realize that these tables work for basic arrhythmias, but not for all complex arrhythmias or mixtures of them; they are good for practice. The final diagnosis, however, depends on the reader's understanding of the "rules" for a specific arrhythmia that were discussed in Chapter 7. It is necessary to memorize the rules, then look for the clues available on each rhythm strip and compare them with the rules. We will briefly review characteristics of four major categories of arrhythmias and three classes of AV block (Table 10–3) at this time. In general, when the QRS duration is not wide, a supraventricular rhythm (sinus, atrial, or AV nodal rhythm) is present. When the QRS duration is wide, either ventricular arrhythmia or supraventricular rhythm with ventricular conduction disturbances (BBB, WPW syndrome, etc.) is present.

TABLE 10–3.
The "Rules" of Major Arrhythmias and AV Blocks

Arrhythmias	
Sinus:	P waves of normal shape (or normal P-axis) in front of each QRS complex, with a regular PR interval
Atrial:	P waves of unusual shape, abnormal number of P waves per QRS complex, or absent P waves
Nodal:	P waves may be absent or, if present, occur after the QRS complex and are inverted
Ventricular:	Wide, bizarre-looking QRS complexes
Atrioventricular blocks	
First degree:	Simple prolongation of PR intervals
Second degree:	Some P waves are not followed by QRS complexes
Mobitz I (Wenckebach):	Progressive lengthening of PR interval with eventual dropped QRS complex
Mobitz II:	Some P waves are not conducted, but the conducted beats have normal, constant PR intervals
2:1 or 3:1 AV block:	Every other or every third P wave is conducted
Third degree (or complete):	P waves and QRS complexes are entirely independent; the RR interval is perfectly regular and occurs at a slower rate than the PP interval

In presenting the drill section, we will demonstrate the use of both the rhythm method and the P wave method on four cases. For the next four cases, the readers will be asked to use both methods. For the remainder of the rhythm strips, only the final interpretation and brief comments, if applicable, will be provided. All rhythm strips shown are lead II unless specified; therefore, sinus rhythm is assumed when the P wave is upright.

CASE 1

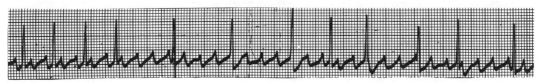

FIG 10–2.
Lead II* rhythm strip from a 14-year-old with congenital mitral stenosis for which a prosthetic valve was inserted at the mitral position.
    *All rhythm strips shown in this chapter are lead II unless otherwise specified.

Rate _90–170_/min   PR ____—____ sec   QRS ____0.06____ sec   QT ____—____ sec
Regularity: _____ Regular (Rate: _____ Normal _____ Fast _____ Slow)
                   _____ Regularly irregular   _x_ Irregularly irregular
                   _____ Single or infrequent   _____ Long pause

Sinus Rhythm: _____ Yes   _x_ No
P waves: _____ Abnormal   _x_ More than   _____ Absent
                   P shape   one P   P waves

Interpretation: Atrial flutter with varying ventricular response.

Interpretation of Case 1

Rhythm Method

The rhythm is irregularly irregular. There are three possibilities (II,B in Table 10–1). It is not ventricular fibrillation because the QRS complex is not wide. It is not atrial fibrillation since the P waves are well formed and the P rate (less than 300) is not fast enough to be fibrillation (400±50). P waves that have "sawtooth" appearance come regularly at a rate of 280 per minute. The number of P waves between R waves is 2 to 4; therefore, 2:1 to 4:1 ventricular response is present.

Interpretation: Atrial flutter with 2:1 to 4:1 ventricular response (i.e., AV block).

P-Wave Method

The rhythm is not sinus. There is more than one P wave between QRS complexes, and the rate is fast (280 per minute) (II,B,1 in Table 10–2). Among three possibilities, the rate is too fast to be atrial tachycardia (240±40), and too slow to be atrial fibrillation (400±50). P waves have the characteristic "sawtooth" appearance of atrial flutter.

Interpretation: Atrial flutter with varying ventricular response.

CASE 2

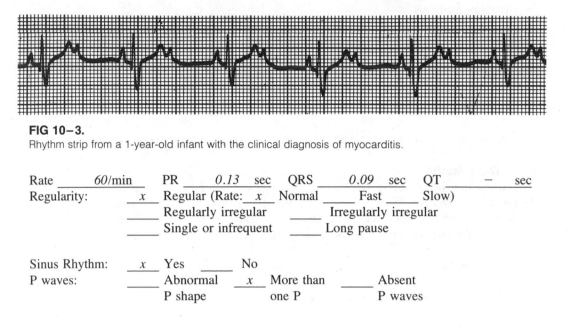

FIG 10–3.
Rhythm strip from a 1-year-old infant with the clinical diagnosis of myocarditis.

Rate _____ 60/min _____ PR _____ 0.13 _____ sec   QRS _____ 0.09 _____ sec   QT _____ − _____ sec

Regularity: __x__ Regular (Rate: __x__ Normal _____ Fast _____ Slow)

                     _____ Regularly irregular   _____ Irregularly irregular

                     _____ Single or infrequent   _____ Long pause

Sinus Rhythm: __x__ Yes   _____ No

P waves: _____ Abnormal   __x__ More than   _____ Absent
                            P shape   one P   P waves

Interpretation: 2:1 second-degree AV block.

Interpretation of Case 2

Rhythm Method

The rhythm is regular with normal heart rate (I,A in Table 10–1). There are two P waves between QRS complexes; therefore, the rhythm is not regular sinus rhythm, but judging from the upright P wave in lead II, the pacemaker site may still be the sinus node. There are four possibilities under I,A,2 in Table 10–1. It is not ectopic atrial rhythm (because P waves are upright in lead II), accelerated AV nodal rhythm (because P waves are present with normal PR interval), or artificial ventricular pacemaker (because no electronic spikes are seen). Only every other P wave gets conducted (second-degree AV block), and the atrial rate (144 per minute) is in the normal range for a 1-year-old infant.

Interpretation: 2:1 second-degree AV block.

P-Wave Method

There are two P waves between QRS complexes; therefore, it is not regular sinus rhythm, but because the P wave is upright in lead II, the pacemaker may still be the sinus node. The atrial rate of 144 per minute is normal for a 1-year-old infant (II,B,2 in Table 10–2). Therefore, AV block is present.

Interpretation: 2:1 second-degree AV block.

CASE 3

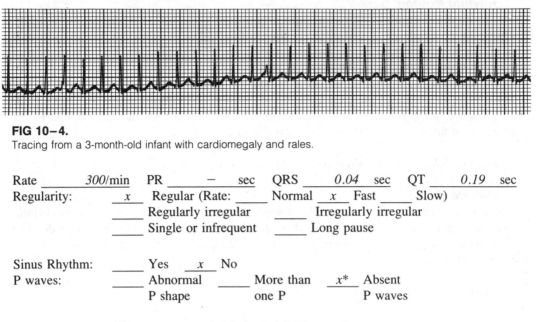

FIG 10–4.
Tracing from a 3-month-old infant with cardiomegaly and rales.

Rate _____*300*/min   PR _____ – _____ sec   QRS _____ *0.04* _____ sec   QT _____ *0.19* _____ sec
Regularity: _*x*_ Regular (Rate: _____ Normal _*x*_ Fast _____ Slow)
                   _____ Regularly irregular   _____ Irregularly irregular
                   _____ Single or infrequent   _____ Long pause

Sinus Rhythm: _____ Yes _*x*_ No
P waves: _____ Abnormal   _____ More than   _*x**_ Absent
                         P shape   one P   P waves

              (*P waves are probably buried in T waves)

Interpretation: Supraventricular tachycardia, probably reciprocating AV tachycardia.

Interpretation of Case 3

Rhythm Method

Regular rhythm with rapid rate is present (I,B in Table 10–1). One finds three possibilities: sinus tachycardia, supraventricular tachycardia, and ventricular tachycardia. Ventricular tachycardia can be easily dismissed because the QRS duration is normal. It is not sinus tachycardia because the rate is too fast; the rate in sinus tachycardia does not exceed 210 per minute. It is supraventricular tachycardia because the QRS duration is normal.

Interpretation: Supraventricular tachycardia. It is unlikely to be nodal tachycardia at this rate, and ectopic atrial tachycardia is less frequent than reciprocating AV tachycardia.

P-Wave Method

There is no visible P wave in front of the QRS complex; therefore, the rhythm is probably not sinus, although at this rate the P wave will be buried in the T wave no matter what the mechanism. However, the rate is too rapid to be sinus in origin. The rhythm is steady or constant, rather than infrequent. Under II,C,2 in Table 10–2, there are six possibilities. Ventricular arrhythmias (ventricular tachycardia and idioventricular rhythm) are immediately dismissed because the QRS duration is not prolonged. The rate is too fast for nodal rhythm (40 to 60 per minute) or accelerated nodal rhythm (60 to 120 per minute). In atrial fibrillation, the rhythm is characteristically "irregularly irregular"; therefore, it is not atrial fibrillation.

Interpretation: Supraventricular tachycardia.

CASE 4

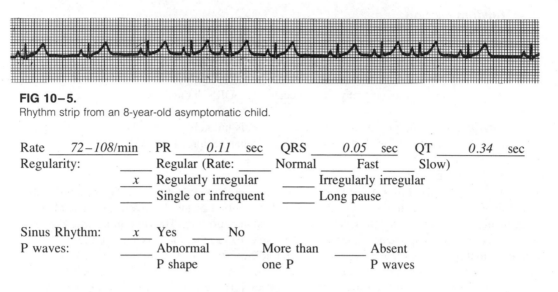

FIG 10–5.
Rhythm strip from an 8-year-old asymptomatic child.

Rate ___72–108___/min   PR ___0.11___ sec   QRS ___0.05___ sec   QT ___0.34___ sec
Regularity: _____ Regular (Rate: _____ Normal _____ Fast _____ Slow)
                     __x__ Regularly irregular   _____ Irregularly irregular
                     _____ Single or infrequent   _____ Long pause

Sinus Rhythm: __x__ Yes   _____ No
P waves: _____ Abnormal   _____ More than   _____ Absent
                           P shape   one P   P waves

Interpretation: Sinus arrhythmia.

Interpretation of Case 4

Rhythm Method

Regularly irregular rhythm is present, with cyclic variation in the heart rate at approximately respiratory rate (II,A in Table 10–1). Upon review of the list, one can exclude Wenckebach block (because no nonconducted P waves are seen) and bigeminal or trigeminal beats. P waves are present before each QRS complex and the P wave is upright in lead II, satisfying criteria for sinus rhythm.

Interpretation: Sinus arrhythmia.

P-Wave Method

All QRS complexes are preceded by P waves of the same morphology and the P waves are upright in lead II, indicating sinus rhythm. The rhythm varies cyclically (arrhythmia).

Interpretation: Sinus arrhythmia.

CASE 5

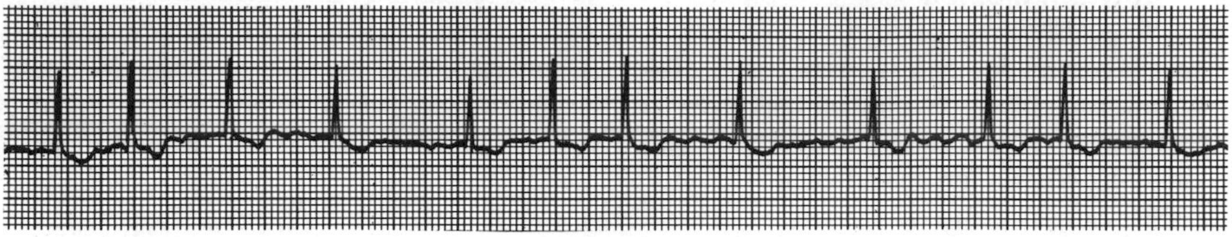

FIG 10-6.
Rhythm strip from a 42-year-old woman with known rheumatic heart disease.

Rate _____ /min PR _____ sec QRS _____ sec QT _____ sec

Regularity: _____ Regular (Rate: _____ Normal _____ Fast _____ Slow)

_____ Regularly irregular _____ Irregularly irregular

_____ Single or infrequent _____ Long pause

Sinus Rhythm: _____ Yes _____ No

P waves: _____ Abnormal _____ More than _____ Absent
P shape one P P waves

*Interpretation:*_____

Interpretation of Case 5

The rhythm is irregularly irregular (II,B in Table 10–1). Ventricular fibrillation can be easily ruled out by the normal QRS complexes. Characteristic "sawtooth" atrial waves of atrial flutter are suggested in short segments only. Irregularly irregular rhythm is characteristic of atrial fibrillation.

Sinus rhythm is not present. Instead, there is more than one P wave seen between some QRS complexes (II,B in Table 10–2). In other areas, the atrial activity appears to have small irregular deflections, characteristic of atrial fibrillation.

Interpretation: Atrial fibrillation.

CASE 6

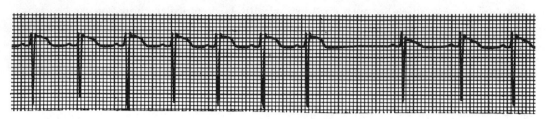

FIG 10–7.
Tracing from an 11-year-old boy with Down's syndrome, endocardial cushion defect, and severe pulmonary hypertension.

Rate _____ /min   PR _____ sec   QRS _____ sec   QT _____ sec
Regularity: _____ Regular (Rate: _____ Normal _____ Fast _____ Slow)
               _____ Regularly irregular   _____ Irregularly irregular
               _____ Single or infrequent   _____ Long pause

Sinus Rhythm: _____ Yes   _____ No
P waves: _____ Abnormal   _____ More than   _____ Absent
               P shape   one P   P waves

*Interpretation:*_____

Interpretation of Case 6

There is one long pause (III in Table 10–1). The pause is interrupted by a sinus beat with regular PR interval. The diagnosis is sinus pause. When there is a long pause like this, one should look for a nonconducted premature atrial contraction (PAC) by carefully inspecting the T wave before the pause for a P′ wave. There is no such wave in this case.

Sinus rhythm is present during most of the record (I in Table 10–2). There is a long pause followed by a sinus beat (with a regular PR interval). The ST-T region following the last normal QRS complex is unaltered (no evidence of nonconducted PAC).

Interpretation: Sinus pause.

CASE 7

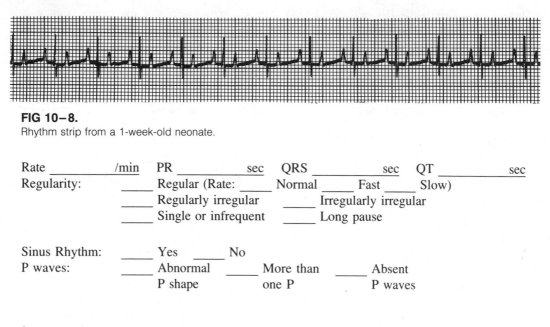

FIG 10–8.
Rhythm strip from a 1-week-old neonate.

Rate _____ /min   PR _____ sec   QRS _____ sec   QT _____ sec
Regularity: _____ Regular (Rate: _____ Normal _____ Fast _____ Slow)
                    _____ Regularly irregular   _____ Irregularly irregular
                    _____ Single or infrequent   _____ Long pause

Sinus Rhythm: _____ Yes   _____ No
P waves: _____ Abnormal   _____ More than   _____ Absent
                    P shape   one P   P waves

*Interpretation:*_____

Interpretation of Case 7

Regular rhythm with normal QRS rate for age (124 per minute) is present, but it is not regular sinus rhythm because there are two P waves between each R wave (I,A,2 in Table 10–1). Every other P wave gets conducted with a regular PR interval (second-degree AV block). The atrial rate is 248 per minute, too fast to be sinus tachycardia, but compatible with atrial tachycardia. Reciprocating AV tachycardia would, by definition, have a 1:1 response.

There are two P waves between QRS complexes (II,B in Table 10–2), and the P rate (248 per minute) is too fast (II,B,1 in Table 10–2) for sinus tachycardia and too slow for atrial flutter. Every other P waves gets conducted and the PR interval for the conducted beat is normal (second-degree AV block).

Interpretation: 2:1 second-degree AV block with ectopic atrial tachycardia. Right atrial hypertrophy is suggested by a 3-mm P wave.

CASE 8

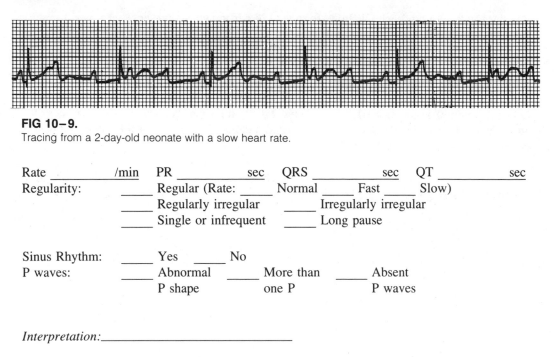

FIG 10−9.
Tracing from a 2-day-old neonate with a slow heart rate.

Rate _____ /min   PR _____ sec   QRS _____ sec   QT _____ sec

Regularity: _____ Regular (Rate: _____ Normal _____ Fast _____ Slow)

                   _____ Regularly irregular   _____ Irregularly irregular

                   _____ Single or infrequent   _____ Long pause

Sinus Rhythm: _____ Yes   _____ No

P waves: _____ Abnormal   _____ More than   _____ Absent

                         P shape   one P   P waves

*Interpretation:*_____

Interpretation of Case 8

The rhythm is regular with the QRS rate of 60 per minute, which is too slow for a normal neonate (I,C in Table 10–1). It is not sinus rhythm because there is more than one P wave in front of the QRS complex and the PR interval is variable. It is not idioventricular rhythm because the QRS duration is normal and the rate is not slow enough. Therefore, it is most likely AV nodal rhythm with complete AV block.

There is more than one P wave between QRS complexes, and the rate is not fast (II,B,2 in Table 10–2); therefore, either second-degree or complete AV block is the diagnosis. The PR interval varies cycle to cycle, indicating a random relationship between the P wave and the QRS complex. The RR interval is perfectly regular. The QRS duration is normal, indicating the complete AV block is above the level of the bifurcation of the bundle of His.

Interpretation: Complete AV block of suprahisian type (AV nodal rhythm with complete AV block).

CASE 9

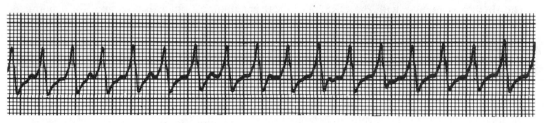

FIG 10–10.
Tracing from an 8-year-old child who had corrective surgery for tetralogy of Fallot, with resulting aneurysm of the right ventricular outflow tract.

CASE 10

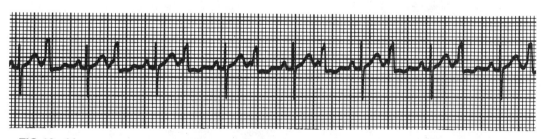

FIG 10–11.
Tracing from a 12-year-old child with appendicitis, who was noted to have irregular heart beats.

Interpretation of Case 9

Interpretation: Ventricular tachycardia.

Comments: The rhythm is regular and the heart rate is rapid (176 per minute). The QRS duration is wide with no regular preceding P wave, suggesting ventricular arrhythmia. One can "walk out" the P waves (see Fig 10–12), indicating an atrial rate of 94 per minute. The independence of atrial and ventricular complexes is characteristic of ventricular tachycardia.

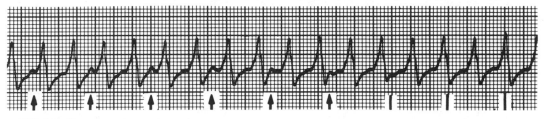

FIG 10–12.
The position of P waves are marked on Figure 10–10.

Interpretation of Case 10

Interpretation: Sinus tachycardia with ventricular bigeminy.

Comments: Regularly irregular rhythm is present with the abnormal beat coming every other beat (bigeminy). The abnormal ventricular beats are premature and have a wide QRS duration. The abnormal beats do have a P wave in front of them (see Fig 10–13), but the PR interval is only 0.05 second, indicating that the complex is a fusion beat between the P and abnormal QRS. When one inspects the P waves, including those marked by arrows in Figure 10–13, one finds the PP interval to be quite regular, with an atrial rate of 166 (sinus tachycardia) in contrast to the prematurity of every other QRS complex, which is abnormally wide.

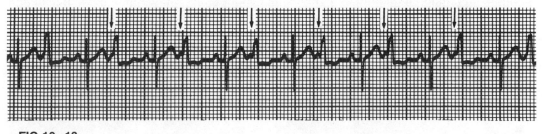

FIG 10–13.
The position of P waves in front of the ventricular arrhythmias is marked by arrows in Figure 10–11.

CASE 11

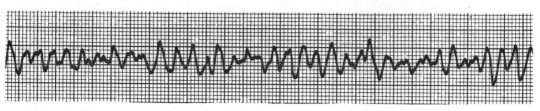

FIG 10–14.
Rhythm strip obtained in the operating room from a 9-month-old infant who was undergoing surgery for tetralogy of Fallot.

CASE 12

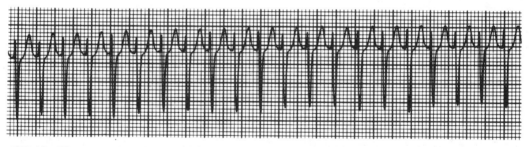

FIG 10–15.
Lead I rhythm strip from a 5-day-old premature infant with tachycardia.

CASE 13

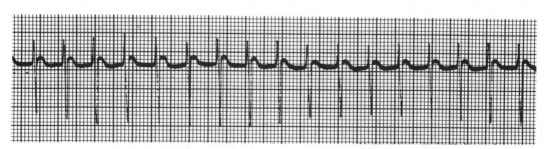

FIG 10–16.
Rhythm strip from a 3-month-old male infant with signs of congestive heart failure.

Interpretation of Case 11

Interpretation: Ventricular fibrillation.

Comments: Note the bizarre QRS complex of varying size and morphology. This arrhythmia requires immediate action. Compare this record with other strips of ventricular fibrillation and realize that QRS morphology varies (see Fig 10–35).

Interpretation of Case 12

Interpretation: Supraventricular tachycardia, probably reciprocating AV tachycardia.

Comments: Note that regularly regular tachycardia (240 per minute) with no visible P waves. This form of tachycardia requires attention, but this is not as urgent as ventricular fibrillation.

Interpretation of Case 13

Interpretation: Supraventricular tachycardia, possibly nodal tachycardia.

Comments: Similar to Figure 10–15, except for the relatively less prominent T waves and slower heart rate (188 per minute).

CASE 14

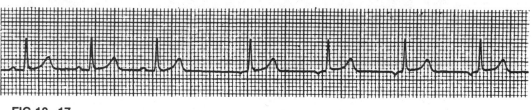

FIG 10–17.
Tracing from an asymptomatic 14-year-old.

CASE 15

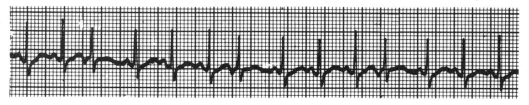

FIG 10–18.
Tracing from a 2-month-old asymptomatic infant.

CASE 16

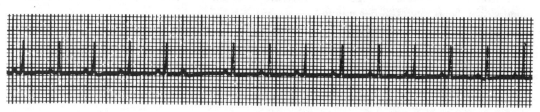

FIG 10–19.
Tracing from a 2-day-old newborn infant with occasional irregular heart beat.

Interpretation of Case 14

Interpretation: Ectopic atrial rhythm.

Comments: The first three cycles are sinus mechanism with a rate of 88 beats per minute. The fourth QRS complex is preceded by an inverted P wave which came later than anticipated time. The sinus node failed to fire and an ectopic focus in the atrium took over the pacemaker activity. The ectopic atrial rate is 75 beats per minute.

Interpretation of Case 15

Interpretation: Premature atrial contractions (PACs).

Comments: There are three premature contractions preceding normal QRS complexes. These premature beats have inverted P waves in front of the QRS complex, which differentiate these from nodal premature beats.

Interpretation of Case 16

Interpretation: Nonconducted PAC.

Comments: Although not common, one should look for a nonconducted PAC when there is a long pause, which could be erroneously read as sinus pause. Note a premature P' wave following the fifth QRS complex. The flat T waves are not abnormal in a newborn infant.

CASE 17

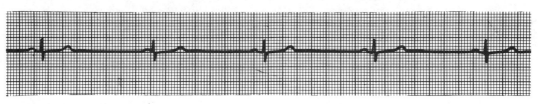

FIG 10–20.
Tracing from a 14-year-old boy in whom sinus node dysfunction developed following repair of a sinus venosus atrial septal defect.

CASE 18

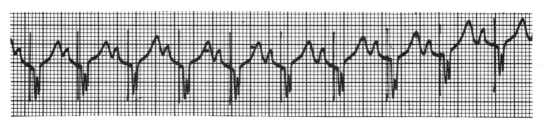

FIG 10–21.
Tracing from a 2-year-old child who developed surgically induced complete heart block, for which an artificial ventricular pacemaker was implanted.

CASE 19

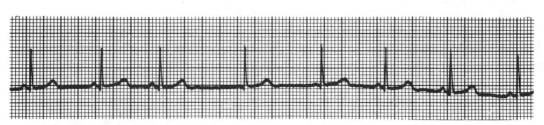

FIG 10–22.
Tracing from a 12-year-old asymptomatic boy.

Interpretation of Case 17

Interpretation: Marked sinus bradycardia, and AV nodal escape beat (the second QRS complex).

Comments: A profound sinus bradycardia is present with the atrial and ventricular rate of 40 per minute (or PP and RR interval of 1.48 sec). The second QRS complex is not a sinus beat; the PR interval for this cycle is much shorter than the PR interval of the other cycles. There was a further slowing of the atrial rate to 38 per minute (or PP interval of 1.58 sec) resulting in a nodal escape beat; the second P-QRS complex represents a fusion beat.

Interpretation of Case 18

Interpretation: P-wave triggered implanted ventricular pacemaker.

Comments: Note the vertical electronic spikes which start ventricular depolarization. The QRS duration is wide as expected. The PR interval has been programmed to be 0.16 second. In this type of pacemaker, the rate of ventricular pacing varies with the rate of the patient's own P wave.

Interpretation of Case 19

Interpretation: Wandering atrial pacemaker.

Comments: There is a *gradual* change in the morphology of the P wave over four cycles. If the P wave shape changes suddenly in one cycle and returns to the original P shape, it is not wandering atrial pacemaker, but is more likely ectopic premature beat. The phasic variation in the heart rate can occur as in sinus arrhythmia.

CASE 20

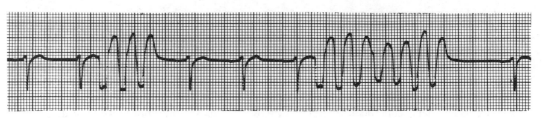

FIG 10–23.
Random lead obtained in the operating room from a 2-year-old child with ventricular septal defect and pulmonary artery banding.

CASE 21

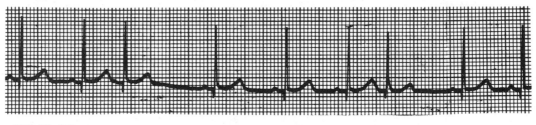

FIG 10–24.
Tracing from a 10-year-old girl with no heart disease.

CASE 22

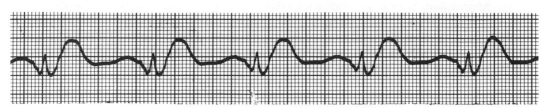

FIG 10–25.
Tracing from an 8-year-old child with severe renal failure.

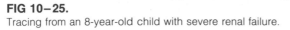

Interpretation of Case 20

Interpretation: Short runs of ventricular tachycardia.

Comments: P waves are not well defined, but this is not lead II, making it difficult to determine sinus versus nonsinus rhythm. Immediate treatment with antiarrhythmic agent such as lidocaine is indicated, followed by a search for the cause.

Interpretation of Case 21

Interpretation: Premature nodal contractions.

Comments: There are two premature beats with normal QRS duration. There appears to be a small upright P wave in front of the third QRS complex, suggesting an ectopic atrial contraction, but there is a compensatory pause following the QRS, suggesting that the sinus node fired on time but the P wave is buried in the T following the premature nodal contraction. No P wave is present in front of the seventh QRS complex, confirming AV nodal origin of both premature beats.

Interpretation of Case 22

Interpretation: Intraventricular block compatible with severe hyperkalemia.

Comments: The QRS duration is markedly increased with slurring throughout the duration of the QRS complex. The heart rate is slow (53 per minute). The P wave is wide and the T wave tall and wide.

CASE 23

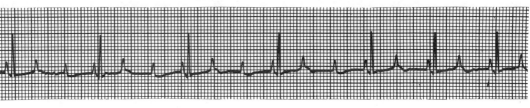

FIG 10–26.
Tracing from a 3-day-old neonate born to a morphine-addicted mother.

CASE 24

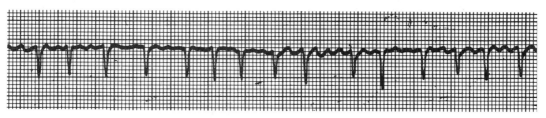

FIG 10–27.
Tracing from a healthy-looking newborn infant with a rapid and variable heart rate.

CASE 25

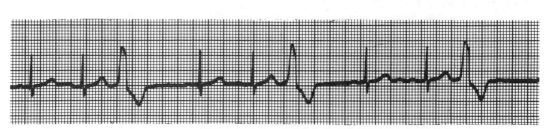

FIG 10–28.
Rhythm strip from a 14-year-old asymptomatic girl.

Interpretation of Case 23

Interpretation: 2:1 and 3:1 second-degree AV block.

Comments: There are two to three P waves between QRS complexes that are normal in duration. The atrial rate is 170 per minute. The QRS rate is much slower. The PR interval for conducted beats appears to be only 0.07 second, and is too short considering the obvious evidence of slowed AV conduction. It is likely that the conducted atrial beat is the one before, with a PR of 0.39 second.

Interpretation of Case 24

Interpretation: Atrial flutter/fibrillation.

Comments: The rhythm is irregularly irregular, a characteristic feature of atrial fibrillation. There are areas where definite "F" waves are seen and other areas where no P waves are seen. These patients may have an underlying disorder of sick sinus syndrome and deserve careful follow-up after conversion.

Interpretation of Case 25

Interpretation: Ventricular trigeminy.

Comments: The abnormal rhythm has a wide QRS complex (arrhythmia of ventricular origin) and comes every third beat. The beat following the ventricular extrasystole occurs at an interval greater than the normal RR interval, indicating a compensatory pause, a characteristic of PVCs.

CASE 26

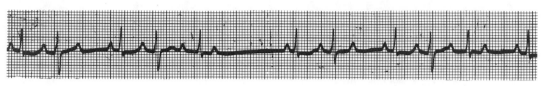

FIG 10−29.
Rhythm strip from an 8-year-old boy with rheumatic myocarditis.

CASE 27

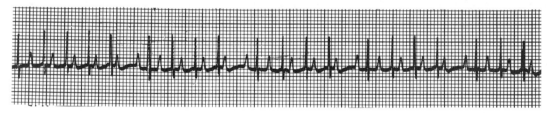

FIG 10−30.
Tracing from a 3-day-old female neonate who received digoxin for congenital atrial tachycardia.

Interpretation of Case 26

Interpretation: Mobitz type I (Wenckebach) second-degree AV block, sinus pause.

Comments: There is gradual lengthening of the PR interval with eventual nonconducted P wave. For example, the PR interval for the third QRS complex is 0.16 second, that for the fourth QRS complex is 0.24, and that for the fifth QRS is 0.28. The P wave following the fifth QRS does not get conducted with a resulting long pause, exaggerated by a sinus pause. (The PP interval doubles between the fifth and sixth R waves.) The conduction ratio in this strip is 3:2, 4:3, 3:2, 4:3, etc. Note that aberrant conduction in the second beat of each Wenckebach cycle.

Interpretation of Case 27

Interpretation: Mobitz type I second-degree AV block, ectopic atrial tachycardia.

Comments: There are characteristics of Wenckebach phenomenon. The conduction ratio is 5:4 with the exception of the first group. The atrial rate is 235 per minute and is too fast to be sinus tachycardia, and fast enough to be atrial tachycardia. The lack of 1:1 response rules out reciprocating AV tachycardia. The initial goal of therapy for atrial tachycardia is to produce enough AV nodal block to lower the ventricular rate. The ventricular rate is still too fast.

CASE 28

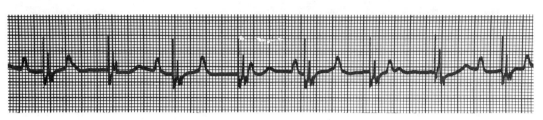

FIG 10–31.
Tracing from a 6-year-old girl with congenital heart block.

CASE 29

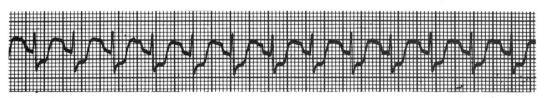

FIG 10–32.
Tracing obtained shortly after a successful cardiopulmonary resuscitation on a 4-year-old child.

CASE 30

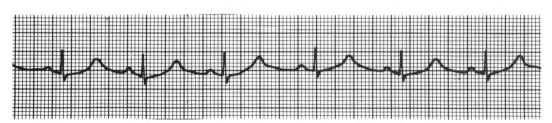

FIG 10–33.
Tracing from the mother of a child with symptomatic Romano-Ward syndrome (syncopal episodes). The mother was asymptomatic.

Interpretation of Case 28

Interpretation: Fixed-rate ventricular pacemaker, complete heart block, and right atrial hypertrophy.

Comments: Vertical electronic spikes depolarize the ventricle with resulting wide QRS complex at a rate of 72 per minute. Tall P waves (RAH) are randomly related to the QRS complexes. The P rate is slightly variable, but is approximately 108 per minute.

Interpretation of Case 29

Interpretation: Sinus tachycardia with ST segment depression.

Comments: The ventricular rate is about 150 per minute. On a quick glance it suggests ventricular tachycardia. However, there are two findings that suggest this to be sinus tachycardia with ST segment depression: (1) the QRS duration appears wide because of pathologic ST segment shift, and (2) one sees a slight distortion of the T wave, suggestive of a P wave, most marked on T waves in front of the first, fourth, and seventh QRS complexes. The PR interval for the fourth beat is approximately 0.12 second.

Interpretation of Case 30

Interpretation: Prolonged QT interval.

Comments: Sinus rhythm is present with the heart rate of 68 per minute. The QT interval (0.48) is abnormally long without including what appeared to be the U wave. The ULN of QT interval for the heart rate is 0.40. The QTc is 0.55, compared to the ULN of 0.44.

CASE 31

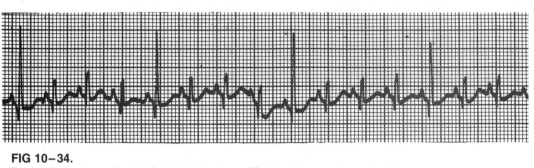

FIG 10–34.
Tracing from a 4-month-old infant with tetralogy of Fallot and severe hypoxic spells.

CASE 32

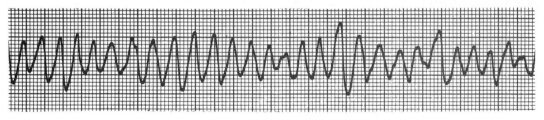

FIG 10–35.
Random lead obtained intraoperatively from a 16-month-old infant with ventricular septal defect.

CASE 33

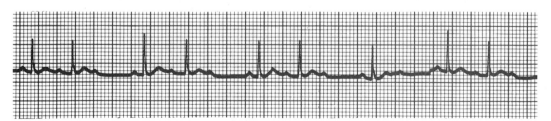

FIG 10–36.
Tracing from a 10-year-old child with recurrent attacks of rheumatic fever with worsening of congestive heart failure. He had involvement of both the mitral and aortic valves.

Interpretation of Case 31

Interpretation: Sinus tachycardia. Respiratory variations in QRS voltage.

Comments: The rhythm is regular and remains sinus at the rate of 166 per minute. Every fourth beat shows tall QRS complex, but the PR interval remains the same. The rate of the large voltage beats is 41 per minute, which coincides with the rate of respiration.

Interpretation of Case 32

Interpretation: Ventricular fibrillation.

Comments: In the first half of the strip, the QRS complex is fairly well organized, suggesting ventricular tachycardia deteriorating to ventricular fibrillation.

Interpretation of Case 33

Interpretation: Mobitz type I (Wenckebach) second-degree AV block.

Comments: In this tracing, the conduction ratio is mostly 3:2, with the exception of one cycle (the third QRS complex from the end) that shows 2:1 conduction ratio.

CASE 34

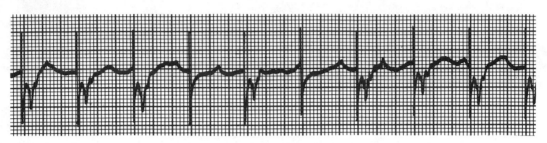

FIG 10–37.
Tracing from a 2-year-old boy who had repair of a VSD and was on a temporary ventricular epicardial pacemaker.

CASE 35

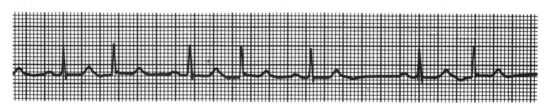

FIG 10–38.
Tracing from a 6-year-old child who had repair of a secundum atrial septal defect.

Interpretation of Case 34

Interpretation: Intermittent failure of fixed-rate ventricular pacemaker to capture and complete heart block.

Comments: The pacemaker rate is set at 100 per minute. The fourth and sixth electronic spikes are not followed by ventricular complexes (wide negative deflection). When one "walks out" the P wave, the atrial rate is approximately 136 per minute. The atrial activity has no fixed relationship to the paced ventricular activity.

Interpretation of Case 35

Interpretation: Frequent ectopic atrial contractions, with occasional failure of AV conduction (non-conducted PAC), and first-degree AV block.

Comments: The second, fourth, and seventh QRS complexes occur prematurely with inverted P waves (PACs). No definite P wave is seen before the fourth QRS complex, suggesting possible nodal premature beat, but the timing similarity argues that all three represent PACs. There is a long pause between the fifth and sixth QRS complexes, and there appears to be an inverted P wave following the T wave of the fifth QRS complex, indicating a non-conducted PAC. Prolongation of PR interval for sinus beat is present.

CASE 36

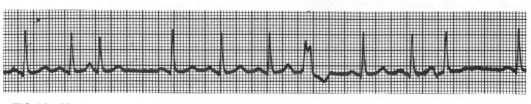

FIG 10–39.
Tracing from a 13-year-old girl with the clinical diagnosis of appendicitis. No evidence of structural heart defect was present.

CASE 37

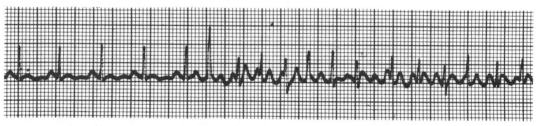

FIG 10–40.
Tracing from a newborn infant with tachycardia.

CASE 38

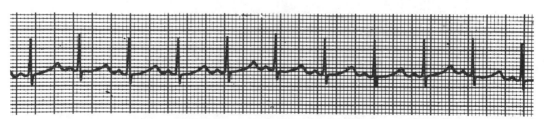

FIG 10–41.
Tracing from an infant of a diabetic mother.

Interpretation of Case 36

Interpretation: Multifocal PACs, and one premature ventricular contraction (PVC).

Comments: The third and the tenth QRS complexes occur prematurely with normal QRS duration (supraventricular). The third QRS complex appears to have an upright P wave in front of it, distorting the T wave, and the tenth QRS complex is preceded by an inverted P wave. The seventh QRS complex is a PVC. There is a sinus pause after PACs, creating an RR interval that is greater than that seen with the compensatory pause of a PVC.

Interpretation of Case 37

Interpretation: Atrial flutter with varying ventricular response.

Comments: Sinus rhythm is present with the heart rate of 136 per minute for the first five cycles. The sixth QRS complex is a premature atrial contraction. This is followed by atrial flutter (approximately 420 per minute) with varying ventricular response; the ventricular rate is approximately 180 per minute.

Interpretation of Case 38

Interpretation: Regular sinus rhythm, and long QT interval suggestive of hypocalcemia.

Comments: The heart rate (115 per minute) is normal for a neonate. The QT interval (0.36) is abnormally long for the heart rate (ULN = 0.33), or the QTc is approximately 0.50. The ST segment appears particularly prolonged, suggesting hypocalcemia, a common finding in an infant of a diabetic mother.

CASE 39

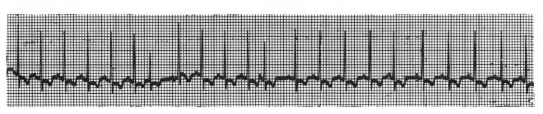

FIG 10–42.
Tracing from a 6-month-old infant with severe congestive heart failure from a large VSD and coarctation of the aorta. The infant was receiving digoxin.

CASE 40

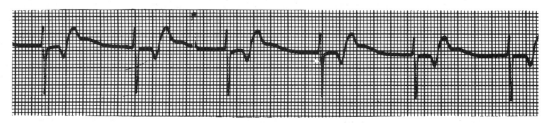

FIG 10–43.
Tracing from a 4-year-old girl with polysplenia syndrome.

CASE 41

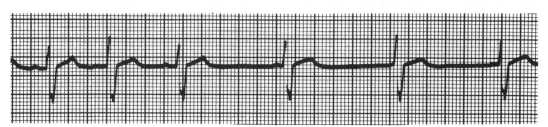

FIG 10–44.
Tracing from a 12-year-old boy who had the Mustard operation for complete transposition of the great arteries during early childhood.

Interpretation of Case 39

Interpretation: Premature nodal and atrial contractions.

Comments: The underlying rhythm is sinus with upright P waves (but with inverted T waves). There are two premature beats. The first premature beat (the seventh QRS) does not show a P wave, suggesting a premature nodal beat. The second premature beat (the 12th QRS) shows an upright slightly different P wave, suggesting a premature atrial contraction, although both premature beats appear to be followed by a compensatory pause of precisely the same duration. These extrasystoles may be signs of digitalis toxicity.

Interpretation of Case 40

Interpretation: Sinus arrest, and AV nodal rhythm with retrogradely conducted P waves.

Comments: There is no P wave in front of the QRS. The ventricular rate is 55 per minute, and the QRS complex is followed by an inverted P wave and an upright T wave. This child has two left atria (with no right atrium) and therefore no sinoatrial node.

Interpretation of Case 41

Interpretation: Sinus pause with AV nodal escape.

Comments: The first three beats are sinus, and the latter three beats the nodal escape beats. The fourth QRS complex represents a fusion beat; the PR interval is much shorter than the PR intervals for the sinus beats.

CASE 42

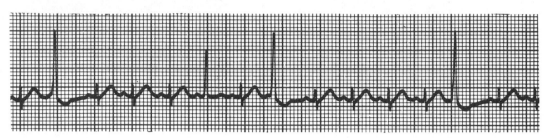

FIG 10−45.
Tracing from a 7-month-old infant with myocarditis.

CASE 43

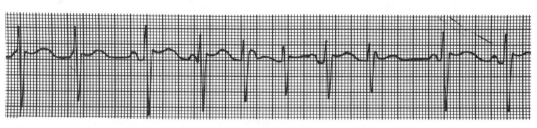

FIG 10−46.
Tracing from a 3-year-old child who was in the immediate postoperative state after the repair of ventricular septal defect. The paper speed was 50/min, twice the usual speed.

CASE 44

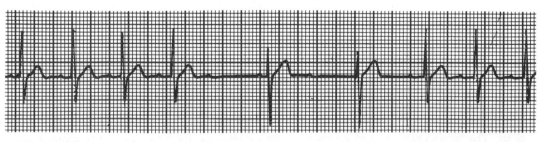

FIG 10−47.
Tracing from an 8-year-old child who had transposition of the great arteries repaired in early childhood.

Interpretation of Case 42

Interpretation: Premature ventricular contractions (PVCs), and one ventricular fusion complex.

Comments: There are three unifocal PVCs with wide QRS complexes and inverted T waves (the second, eighth, and 13th QRS complexes). The sixth QRS complex is slightly taller and different from the sinus QRS complex or the QRS complex of the PVCs. There is a P with slightly shorter PR interval for the sixth QRS complex, suggesting that this P wave was not conducted. This is a ventricular fusion complex.

Interpretation of Case 43

Interpretation: Atrioventricular dissociation due to accelerated rate of AV nodal pacemaker.

Comments: Considering the paper speed of 50 mm/sec, the atrial rate is approximately 160 per minute and regular (see Fig 10–48). The QRS complex is normal, and its rate in the midportion of the tracing is about 230 per minute. The third and last QRS complexes are probably conducted sinus beats.

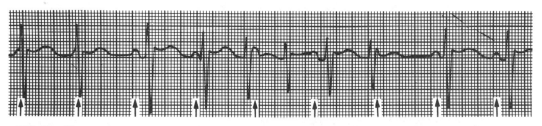

FIG 10–48.
P waves are indicated by *arrows*.

Interpretation of Case 44

Interpretation: Second-degree heart block (Mobitz type II) with AV nodal escape beats.

Comments: The first four beats are sinus rhythm with normal PR interval. The fourth QRS complex is followed by four nonconducted P waves. Three P waves are visible, and the fourth P wave is hidden in the sixth QRS complex (Fig 10–49). During this time, two nodal escape beats occur with altered conduction. The last three QRS complexes are sinus beats.

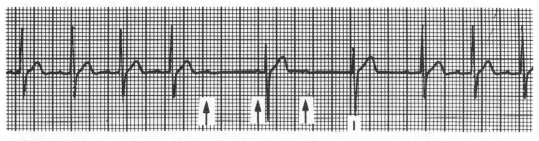

FIG 10–49.
The position of P waves is marked on Figure 10–47.

CASE 45

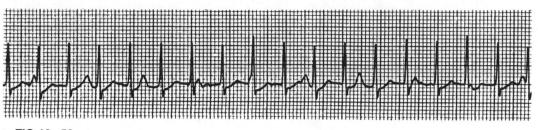

FIG 10–50.
Tracing from a 4-year-old child in postoperative state for transposition of the great arteries.

Interpretation of Case 45

Interpretation: Atrioventricular dissociation due to accelerated AV nodal rate.

Comments: The ventricular rate is 188 beats per minute with normal QRS duration. P waves are not present regularly in front of each QRS complex. On closer inspection, it appears that the P waves come at a slower rate. Using the "walk out" method, one can identify P waves (see Fig 10–51) with a rate of about 100 beats per minute, which is normal rate for a 4-year-old child. Therefore, the AV dissociation is due to accelerated rate of the AV node or junctional tissue (with normal QRS duration).

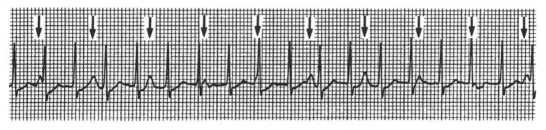

FIG 10–51.
The position of P waves is marked on Fig 10–50.

Appendix

HOW TO AVOID COMMON ERRORS AND ARTIFACTS IN RECORDING

1. Be certain there is a good contact between the skin and the electrode.
2. Attach extremity leads to their respective electrodes to record six limb leads. Errors in connecting electrodes will result in abnormal axes for the P, QRS, and T. Figure A−1 is an example of switching the right and left arm leads.
3. Standardize the machine so that 1 millivolt produces a deflection of 1 centimeter, and record the calibration mark. Improper standardization or failure to mark the calibration factor will result in false-negative or false-positive diagnoses of ventricular or atrial hypertrophy.
4. If using (old) ECG machine with manual dial, turn the dial to the V position to record the precordial leads. Failure to do so will result in precordial leads that are identical to aVF throughout the precordial leads (V1 through V6).
5. There are three important precautions to be kept in mind in recording the precordial leads:
   a. Make sure you start V1 in the fourth intercostal space. If you move one space up (third interspace), you will obtain an ECG showing much smaller voltages (Fig A−2).
   b. Be precise in locating V6. If too close to V5, a larger voltage will be recorded, simulating LVH (see Fig 9−14). If positioned too high, a deep S may be recorded, simulating RVH.
   c. Use a small pediatric chest piece (suction cup) for infants and small children. Preferably use an individual adhesive electrode (without conducting jelly) with a newer type of ECG machine; this will prevent smearing effects of the electrode paste.
   d. If using an old ECG machine, make sure the electrode paste is wiped off before moving to the next location on a small infant. Also make sure that the electrode paste does not form "bridges" with adjacent electrodes. Failure to do so will result in large diphasic QRS deflections, almost identical throughout the precordial leads, which might be interpreted as combined ventricular hypertrophy. Fig A−3 (see Appendix) is an example of this.

Example (Fig A–1)

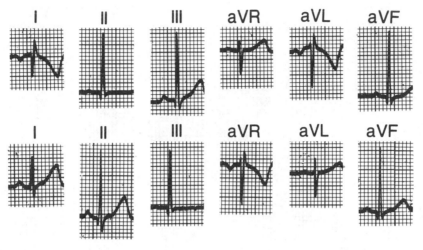

FIG A-1.
Tracing in *top panel* was obtained with patient's right-arm and left-arm electrodes switched. Tracing in *bottom panel* was obtained with electrodes placed correctly.

A clue to this type of technical error is the presence of an abnormal P axis in the right lower quadrant. In a normal child the QRS and T axes will also be in the right lower quadrant. This type of abnormal axis is also seen in mirror-image dextrocardia (see Chap. 8). Note that leads II and III as well as aVR and aVL are interchanged.

Example (Fig A–2)

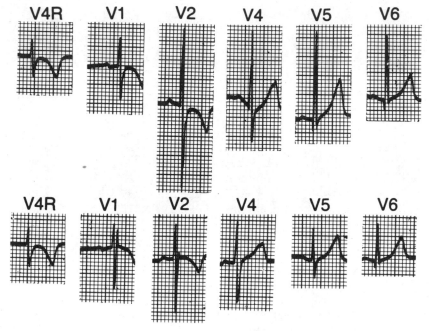

FIG A–2.

Tracing in *top panel* was obtained with precordial leads placed correctly, with the VI lead starting in the fourth intercostal space. Tracing in *bottom panel* was obtained with VI starting one space up, in the third interspace.

Note that the voltages are generally lower in the bottom panel and there is rsr′ pattern in V1 similar to that expected in aVR.

Example (Fig A–3)

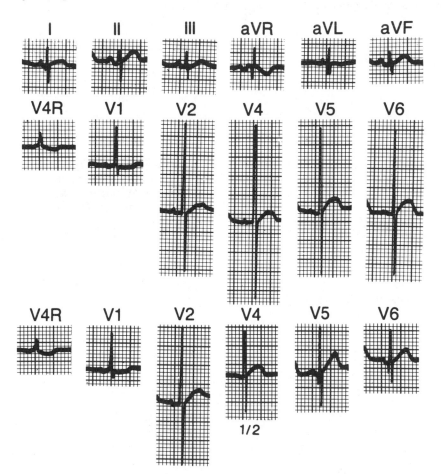

FIG A–3.
Tracing was obtained in infant when electrode paste was not wiped off between V-leads *(second row)*. Tracing in the *third row* was obtained in correct way.

Note that there are large diphasic QRS deflections with poor R/S progression (in the second row). This tracing might have been interpreted as combined ventricular hypertrophy, although that diagnosis is not suggested by the frontal plane. A repeat of the precordial leads (shown in the third row) shows remarkable differences from the original recording. Note the differences in leads V4 through V6. Even though the V1 electrode was not wiped off, there must have been no conductive bridge between the V1 and V2 positions.

TABLE A–1.

Common ECG Manifestations of Some Congenital Heart Defects

Congenital Defects	ECG Findings
Anomalous origin of the left coronary artery from the pulmonary artery (see Fig 6–10)	Myocardial infarction, anterolateral
Anomalous pulmonary venous return	
Total	RAD, RVH, and RAH
Partial	Mild RVH or RBBB
Aortic stenosis	
Mild to moderate	Normal or LVH
Severe	LVH with or without "strain"
Atrial septal defect	
Primum type	Left anterior hemiblock (superior QRS axis)
	rsR′ pattern in V1 and aVR (RBBB or RVH)
	First-degee AV block (>50%)
	Counterclockwise QRS loop in the frontal plane of VCG
Secundum type (see Figs 5-6 and 9–12)	RAD, RVH, or RBBB (rsR′ in V1 and aVR)
	First-degree AV block (10%)
Coarctation of the aorta	
Infants less than 6 months old	RBBB or RVH
Older children	LVH, normal, or RBBB
Common ventricle or single ventricle (see Fig 9–15)	Abnormal Q waves
	Q in V1 and no Q in V6
	No Q in any precordial leads
	Q in all precordial leads
	Stereotype RS complex in most or all precordial leads
	WPW syndome or PAT
	First- or second-degree AV block
Cor triatriatum	Same as for mitral stenosis
Ebstein's anomaly (see Fig 9–1)	RAH, RBBB
	First-degree AV block
	WPW syndrome
	No RVH
Endocardial cushion defect	
Complete (see Fig 9–11)	Left anterior hemiblock (superior QRS axis)
	RVH or CVH, RAH
	First-degree AV block, RBBB
Partial	See ASD, primum type
Endocardial fibroelastosis (see Fig 9–7)	LVH
	Abnormal T waves
	Infarction patterns
Hypoplastic left heart syndrome (aortic and/or mitral atresia)	RVH
Mitral stenosis, congenital or acquired (see Fig 4–4)	RAD, RVH, RAH, LAH (±)
Patent ductus arteriosus	
Small shunt	Normal
Moderate shunt	LVH, LAH (±)
Large shunt (see Fig 4–13)	CVH, LAH
Eisenmenger's syndrome (pulmonary vascular obstructive disease)	RVH or CVH

TABLE A-1 (cont.).

Common ECG Manifestations of Some Congenital Heart Defects

Congenital Defects	ECG Findings
Persistent truncus arteriosus (see Fig 9–9)	LVH or CVH
Pulmonary atresia (with hypoplastic RV) (see Figs 4–3 and 9–2)	LVH
Pulmonary stenosis	
Mild	Normal or mild RVH
Moderate (see Fig 4–10)	RVH
Severe (see Fig 9–13)	RVH with "strain"
	RAH
Pulmonary vascular obstructive disease (Eisenmenger's syndrome) (see Fig 4–13)	RVH or CVH
Tetralogy of Fallot (see Fig 4–8)	RAD
	RVH, moderate or severe
	RAH (±)
D-transposition of the great arteries (complete transposition)	
Intact ventricular septum (see Fig 9–6)	RVH, RAH
VSD and/or PS	CVH, RAH, or CAH
L-transposition of the great arteries ("corrected" transposition) (see Fig 8–7)	AV block, first to third degree
	Atrial arrhythmias (PAT, atrial fibrillation)
	WPW syndrome
	Absent Q in V5 and V6 and qR pattern in V1
	LAH or CAH
Tricuspid atresia (see Fig 9–5)	Left anterior hemiblock (superior QRS axis)
	LVH, RAH
Ventricular septal defect	
Small shunt	Normal
Moderate shunt (see Fig 4–12)	LVH, LAH (±)
Large shunt (see Fig 4–13)	CVH, LAH
Pulmonary vascular obstructive disease (Eisenmenger's syndrome)	RVH

CLASSIFICATION OF CONGENITAL HEART DISEASE ACCORDING TO ECG AND CLINICAL AND PHYSIOLOGIC STATUS

Right Ventricular Abnormalities

Cyanotic Defects (Right-to-Left Shunt)

1. Decreased pulmonary blood flow + RVH
   a. Severe pulmonary stenosis with ventricular septal defect (VSD), i.e., tetralogy of Fallot
   b. Severe pulmonary stenosis with atrial septal defect (ASD), or patent foramen ovale.
   c. Transposition of great arteries with pulmonary stenosis.
   d. Severe pulmonary vascular obstruction ("Eisenmenger's physiology"), with VSD, ASD, PDA, etc.
2. Decreased pulmonary blood flow + RBBB
   a. Ebstein's anomaly (also marked p-pulmonale)
3. Increaed pulmonary blood flow + RVH
   a. "Fetal" coarctation with RV supplying postductal aorta (includes aortic atresia and hypoplastic left heart syndrome).
   b. Total anomalous pulmonary venous return
   c. Transposition of great arteries

Acyanotic Defects

1. Left-to-right shunt + RVH: All left-to-right shunts with moderately increased pressure in RV, secondary to mild pulmonary stenosis or mild increase in pulmonary vascular resistance.
2. Left-to-right shunt + RVH or RBBB: ASD (including partial anomalous pulmonary venous return).
3. No shunts + RVH
   a. Pulmonary stenosis.
   b. Pulmonary hypertension, primary or secondary to mitral stenosis or cor triatriatum.
4. No shunts + RBBB: "Adult type" coarctation in infants.

Left Ventricular Hypertrophy

Cyanotic Defects

1. Decreased pulmonary blood flow: Tricuspid atresia (p-pulmonale).
2. Increased pulmonary blood flow
   a. (Rarely) single ventricle alone or with truncus arteriosus.
   b. Tricuspid atresia with transposition of great arteries.

Acyanotic Defects

1. Left-to-right shunt
   a. VSD.
   b. PDA and other arteriovenous fistulae.
   c. Septum primum ASD with mitral regurgitation (left anterior hemiblock).

2. No shunts
   a. Aortic stenosis.
   b. Aortic regurgitation.
   c. Coarctation of aorta.
   d. Mitral regurgitation.
   e. Primary myocardial diseases (endocardial fibroelastosis).

Combined Ventricular Hypertrophy (Including "Single Ventricle" ECG)

Cyanotic Defects

1. Decreased pulmonary blood flow
   a. Single or common ventricle with pulmonary stenosis and/or transposition of great arteries.
   b. Single ventricle with truncus arteriosus and hypoplastic pulmonary arteries.
2. Increased pulmonary blood flow
   a. Transposition of great arteries with pulmonary hypertension.
   b. Single or common ventricle.
   c. Truncus arteriosus.
   d. VSD with moderate pulmonary stenosis.
   e. Pulmonary atresia with huge PDA.

Acyanotic Defects

1. Left-to-right shunt
   a. Large VSD with mild increase in pulmonary vascular resistance, or moderate pulmonary stenosis.
   b. Large PDA with mild increase in pulmonary vascular resistance.
   c. Endocardial cushion defect, partial or complete.
2. No shunts: Combination of obstructive lesions (e.g., pulmonary stenosis plus aortic stenosis).

TABLES OF NORMAL VALUES

TABLE A-2.

PQ (PR) Interval, With Rate and Age (and Upper Limits of Normal)

Rate	0–1 mo	1–6 mo	6 mo–1 yr	1–3 yr	3–8 yr	8–12 yr	12–16 yr	Adult
<60						0.16(0.18)	0.16(0.19)	0.17(0.21)
60–80					0.15(0.17)	0.15(0.17)	0.15(0.18)	0.16(0.21)
80–100	0.10(0.12)				0.14(0.16)	0.15(0.16)	0.15(0.17)	0.15(0.20)
100–120	0.10(0.12)			(0.15)	0.13(0.16)	0.14(0.15)	0.15(0.16)	0.15(0.19)
120–140	0.10(0.11)	0.11(0.14)	0.11(0.14)	0.12(0.14)	0.13(0.15)	0.14(0.15)		0.15(0.18)
140–160	0.09(0.11)	0.10(0.13)	0.11(0.13)	0.11(0.14)	0.12(0.14)			(0.17)
160–180	0.10(0.11)	0.10(0.12)	0.10(0.12)	0.10(0.12)				
>180	0.09	0.09(0.11)	0.10(0.11)					

Modified from Guntheroth WG: *Pediatric Electrocardiography.* Philadelphia, WB Saunders Co, 1965.

TABLE A-3.

QRS Duration: Average (and Upper Limits) for Age

	0–1 mo	1–6 mo	6 mo–1 yr	1–3 yr	3–8 yr	8–12 yr	12–16 yr	Adult
Seconds	0.05(0.065)	0.05(0.07)	0.05(0.07)	0.06(0.07)	0.07(0.08)	0.07(0.09)	0.07(0.10)	0.08(0.10)

Modified from Guntheroth WG: *Pediatric Electrocardiography.* Philadelphia, WB Saunders Co, 1965. (Used by permission.)

TABLE A-4.

R Voltages According to Lead and Age: Mean (and Upper Limits)*

Lead	0–1 mo	1–6 mo	6 mo–1 yr	1–3 yr	3–8 yr	8–12 yr	12–16 yr	Young Adults
I	4 (8)	7 (13)	8 (16)	8 (16)	7 (15)	7 (15)	6 (13)	6 (13)
II	6 (14)	13 (24)	13 (27)	13 (23)	13 (22)	14 (24)	14 (24)	9 (25)
III	8 (16)	9 (20)	9 (20)	9 (20)	9 (20)	9 (24)	9 (24)	6 (22)
aVR	3 (7)	3 (6)	3 (6)	2 (6)	2 (5)	2 (4)	2 (4)	1 (4)
aVL	2 (7)	4 (8)	5 (10)	5 (10)	3 (10)	3 (10)	3 (12)	3 (9)
aVF	7 (14)	10 (20)	10 (16)	8 (20)	10 (19)	10 (20)	11 (21)	5 (23)
V4R	6 (12)	5 (10)	4 (8)	4 (8)	3 (8)	3 (7)	3 (7)	
V1	15 (25)	11 (20)	10 (20)	9 (18)	7 (18)	6 (16)	5 (16)	3 (14)
V2	21 (30)	21 (30)	19 (28)	16 (25)	13 (28)	10 (22)	9 (19)	6 (21)
V5	12 (30)	17 (30)	18 (30)	19 (36)	21 (36)	22 (36)	18 (33)	12 (33)
V6	6 (21)	10 (20)	13 (20)	12 (24)	14 (24)	14 (24)	14 (22)	10 (21)

S Voltages According to Lead and Age: Mean (and Upper Limits)*

Lead	0–1 mo	1–6 mo	6 mo–1 yr	1–3 yr	3–8 yr	8–12 yr	12–16 yr	Young Adults
I	5 (10)	4 (9)	4 (9)	3 (8)	2 (8)	2 (8)	2 (8)	1 (6)
V4R	4 (9)	4 (12)	5 (12)	5 (12)	5 (14)	6 (20)	6 (20)	
V1	10 (20)	7 (18)	8 (16)	13 (27)	14 (30)	16 (26)	15 (24)	10 (23)
V2	20 (35)	16 (30)	17 (30)	21 (34)	23 (38)	23 (38)	23 (48)	14 (36)
V5	9 (30)	9 (26)	8 (20)	6 (16)	5 (14)	5 (17)	5 (16)	
V6	4 (12)	2 (7)	2 (6)	2 (6)	1 (5)	1 (4)	1 (5)	1 (13)

*Voltages are measured in millimeters, when 1 mV = 10 mm paper.
Modified from Guntheroth WG: *Pediatric Electrocardiography.* Philadelphia, WB Saunders Co, 1965.

TABLE A-5.

Q Voltages According to Lead and Age: Mean (and Upper Limits)*

Lead	0-1 mo	1-6 mo	6 mo-1 yr	1-3 yr	3-8 yr	8-12 yr	12-16 yr	Adult
III	2 (5)	3 (8)	3 (8)	3 (8)	1.5 (6)	1 (5)	1 (4)	0.5 (4)
aVF	2 (4)	2 (5)	2 (6)	1.5 (5)	1 (5)	1 (3)	1 (3)	0.5 (2)
V5	1.5 (5)	1.5 (4)	2 (5)	2 (6)	2 (6)	2 (4.5)	1 (4)	0.5 (3.5)
V6	1.5 (4)	1.5 (4)	2 (5)	2 (4.5)	1.5 (4.5)	1.5 (4)	1 (2.5)	0.5 (3)

*Voltages measured in millimeters, when 1 mV = 10 mm paper.
From Guntheroth WG: *Pediatric Electrocardiography*. Philadelphia, WB Saunders Co, 1965. (Used by permission.)

TABLE A-6.

R/S Ratio According to Age: Mean, Lower, and Upper Limits of Normal

Lead	0-1 mo	1-6 mo	6 mo-1 yr	1-3 yr	3-8 yr	8-12 yr	12-16 yr	Adult
LLN*	0.5	0.3	0.3	0.5	0.1	0.15	0.1	0.0
V1 Mean	1.5	1.5	1.2	0.8	0.65	0.5	0.3	0.3
ULN†	19	S = 0	6	4	2	1	1	1
LLN	0.3	0.3	0.3	0.3	0.05	0.1	0.1	0.1
V2 Mean	1	1.2	1	0.8	0.5	0.5	0.5	0.2
ULN	3	4	4	1.5	1.5	1.2	1.2	2.5
LLN	0.1	1.5	2	3	2.5	4	2.5	2.5
V6 Mean	2	4	6	20	20	20	10	9
ULN	S = 0	S = 0	S = 0	S = 0	S = 0	S = 0	S = 0	S = 0

*Lower limits of normal.
†Upper limits of normal.
Modified from Guntheroth WG: *Pediatric Electrocardiography*. Philadelphia, WB Saunders Co, 1965. (Used by permission.)

TABLE A-7.

Cycle Length, Heart Rate, and Q-T Interval Average (and Upper Limits)

Cycle Length (sec)	Heart Rate (per min)	Average QT (Upper Limit) (sec)	Cycle Length (sec)	Heart Rate (per min)	Average QT (Upper Limit) (sec)
1.50	40	0.45 (0.49)	0.85	70	0.36 (0.38)
1.40	43	0.44 (0.48)	0.80	75	0.35 (0.38)
1.30	46	0.43 (0.47)	0.75	80	0.34 (0.37)
1.25	48	0.42 (0.46)	0.70	86	0.33 (0.36)
1.20	50	0.41 (0.45)	0.65	92	0.32 (0.35)
1.15	52	0.41 (0.45)	0.60	100	0.31 (0.34)
1.10	55	0.40 (0.44)	0.55	109	0.30 (0.33)
1.05	57	0.39 (0.43)	0.50	120	0.28 (0.31)
1.00	60	0.39 (0.42)	0.45	133	0.27 (0.29)
0.95	63	0.38 (0.41)	0.40	150	0.25 (0.28)
0.90	67	0.37 (0.40)	0.35	172	0.23 (0.26)

From Guntheroth WG: *Pediatric Electrocardiography*. Philadelphia, WB Saunders Co, 1965. (Used by permission.)

Answers to Review Questions

CHAPTER 1

1. (A) 82, (B) 128, (C) 155, (D) 64
2. c
3. c
4. P axis = +40 degrees, QRS axis = +60 degrees, T axis = +30 degrees, QRS-T angle = 30 degrees
5. Intermediate
6. a
7. QRSi = +115 degrees, QRSt = −55 degrees
8. True
9. True
10. True
11. True
12. False
13. False
14. False
15. False

CHAPTER 2

1. True
2. False
3. True
4. False
5. False
6. True
7. True
8. True
9. True

CHAPTER 3

1. False
2. True
3. True
4. False
5. False
6. False
7. False
8. True
9. False

CHAPTER 4

1. a, b, c, and d
2. a and b
3. a and b
4. False
5. True
6. False
7. True
8. False
9. True
10. False

CHAPTER 5

1. b
2. b
3. b
4. a

5. d
6. e
7. True
8. True
9. True
10. True
11. True
12. False

CHAPTER 6

1. a
2. a
3. a
4. False
5. True
6. False
7. True
8. True
9. True
10. True
11. False
12. True

CHAPTER 7

1. False
2. True
3. True
4. True
5. False
6. True
7. True
8. True
9. False
10. True
11. True
12. True

CHAPTER 8

1. False
2. True
3. True
4. True

Index